GASTRIC SLEEVE BARIATRIC COOKBOOK FOR BEGINNERS

Easy Guide + 159 Healthy Recipes to Speed Up Your Recovery, Minimize Side Effects and Keep the Weight Off.

Summer Kelly

Table of Contents

Introduction

The gastric sleeve is also often referred to as the vertical sleeve gastrectomy or simply the sleeve gastrectomy has been around for many years, and the procedure is often performed by bariatric surgeons as the first procedure in a two-part weight loss procedure.

In patients who are highly obese with BMI in excess of 60, conventional gastric bypass surgery such as roux-en-y, this poses unacceptably high risks, and so the gastric sleeve is done because this operation can typically be conducted laparoscopically with minimal risk. Instead, a second procedure, such as classical gastric bypass surgery, can be performed when you have lost enough weight.

However, the view of the gastric sleeve has changed in recent years, and it is now primarily being used as a stand-alone operation that can yield outcomes close to those seen with lap band surgery on its own.

The sleeve gastrectomy may be an attractive choice for patients who are worried about lap-band surgery because they are concerned about having a foreign body inserted into their abdomen. Similarly, it also presents an alternative for those patients who are concerned about possible long-term side effects of gastric bypass surgery such as anemia, intestinal obstruction, ulcers, and deficiency of vitamins and proteins, to name a few.

Another group of patients for whom the gastrectomy of the vertical sleeve may be a lifesaver are those persons with an existing medical condition that rule out traditional obesity surgery. For example, patients with Crohn's disease, Lupus, anemia, and a whole array of other medical conditions.

The gastric sleeve is a strictly restricting treatment rather than malabsorption and induces weight loss by regulating how much you can consume. As a purely restrictive form of surgery, weight loss is slower than it would be with bypass operation, but you also avoid many of the side effects and complications associated with a bypass operation. While there are no long-term data yet available for the gastric sleeve as a stand-alone procedure initial reports, indicate that high BMI patients (with a BMI of between 50 and 60) may expect to lose about half their excess weight in the first year following surgery. This percentage increases to more than two-thirds of excess weight for patients with lower BMIs (with a BMI of 30 to 40).

In terms of weight loss surgery, the stomach sleeve fits between the stomach band and the stomach bypass and can be a good choice for patients whose overall health makes stomach bypass surgery inadvisable, and it can produce enough weight loss for many patients to make a very significant difference in their health and lifestyle.

Chapter 1

UNDERSTANDING GASTRIC SLEEVE SURGERY

WHAT IS GASTRIC SLEEVE SURGERY

Vertical sleeve gastrectomy, also known as gastric sleeve surgery, is a process in which the stomach's capacity to hold the food is reduced by 80 percent. In other words, a sleeve is created on the side of the stomach, which receives the food in a small amount; the rest is separated through this surgery. This bariatric procedure is also called weight loss surgery as it is used to induce weight loss through a permanent approach. The following diagram shows how the stomach walls are stitched together to create a separate sleeve for food digestion:

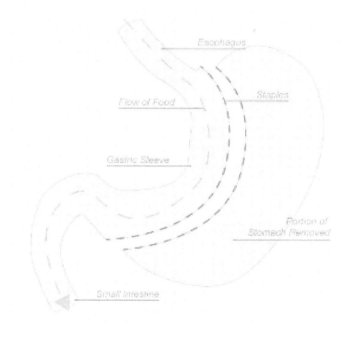

Diagram: Post Gastric Sleeve Surgery Stomach

WHY IS IT NEEDED?

The gastric sleeve surgery is mainly opted to achieve weight loss. This surgery works for people who are sensitive to dietary changes and just can't lose weight through diet control. So, this surgery finds a permanent solution and reduces the stomach size, which automatically cuts down food consumption.

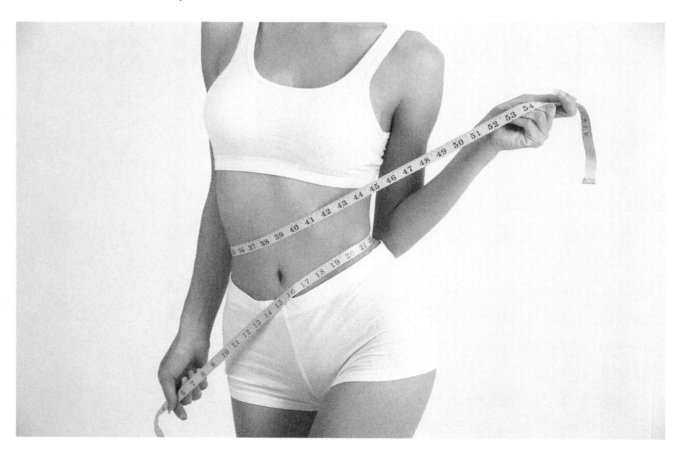

This surgery has given effective results, and within one year of the surgery, people should 70 percent weight loss. By controlling obesity, such individuals were also able to resist diabetes, insulin resistance, sleep apnea, hypertension, joints pain, fatty liver disease, and hyperlipidemia. Excessive hunger sensation is also reduced to a minimum after gastric sleeve surgery.

The procedure is indeed effective, but it works well only when a person changes his dietary habits after the surgery and follows a gastric sleeve diet.

Pre-Surgery Tips:

- Change your diet and switch to a liquid-only diet a week before the surgery.

- If you are a smoker, then stop smoking at least 2 weeks before the surgery to avoid complications.

- Discuss your health condition and post-surgery effects with your doctor before the surgery.

- Clean your kitchen and set up the pantry according to the new lifestyle.

- Increase the protein intake to prepare the body for quick recovery after the surgery.

Post-Surgery Tips

- Switch to the gastric sleeve diet and use more clear liquids right after the surgery.

- Add protein-based supplements and liquids to the diet to ensure quick recovery and healing of the stomach.

- Start with the intake of soft food and gradually switch to the proper meals.

- Stop having heavy, oily food on the table.

- Light exercises and yoga ensure quick recovery, so try some light exercises 2-3 days after the surgery.

- Consult your dietician and the doctor after every week to discuss your diet and changing health conditions.

Chapter 2

GASTRIC SLEEVE DIET

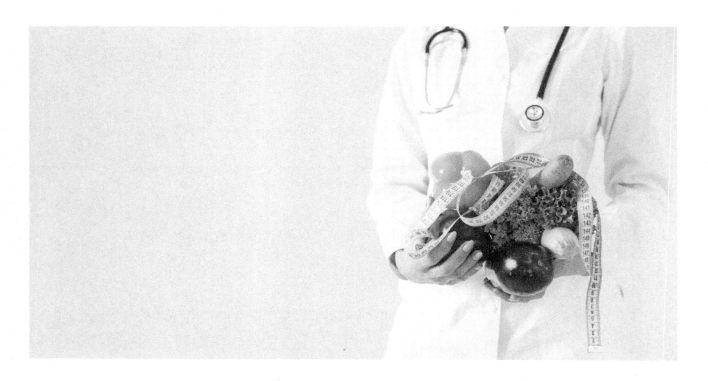

WHAT IS A GASTRIC SLEEVE DIET?

Gastric diet is one of the strict diet plans followed before and after gastric sleeve surgery. It strictly reduces the intake of calories and carbohydrates. These calories and carbohydrates are coming from sweets, pasta, and potatoes. During gastric sleeve diet, you have to consume liquid foods that are low in calories and high in protein. Protein helps to maintain your muscle mass and also helps to maintain your body energy level. Before two days of surgery, you have to switch to a clear liquid diet, such as sugar-free protein shake, decaffeinated coffee or tea, sugar-free popsicles, broth, and water. During the gastric sleeve diet, completely avoid caffeinated and carbonated beverages.

After gastric sleeve surgery, a person must follow a strict diet to recover your body and adjust to the smaller size of your stomach. The person with gastric sleeve surgery eats smaller and more frequent meals for the rest of their lives. The diet plan can be divided into four stages:

STAGE ONE DIET: CLEAR LIQUIDS

This stage is beginning in the first week after your gastric sleeve surgery. In this stage of the diet, only a few ounces of food drinks have been allowed. This will help your stomach heal without getting stretched by foods. The liquid diet includes:

- Water

- Thin soup and broth

- Skim milk

- Decaffeinated coffee and tea

- Sugar-free gelatin and popsicles

- Unsweetened juice.

Avoid sugary liquids during the first week of gastric sleeve surgery. Consuming sugary drinks may lead to raising digestive problems and occurs negative side effect on surgery. Also, avoid carbonated and caffeinated beverages. During the first week of surgery, always stay your body hydrated, just remember only drink a small amount of liquid at a time.

STAGE TWO DIET: PROTEIN-RICH LIQUIDS

The stage two begins after five days of gastric sleeve surgery. During this stage, you have to allow consuming protein-rich shake and more liquids like Skimmed milk, unsweetened, and blended fruit juice. During this stage, you experience an increase in your appetite appetite, but you have to stick to your diet plan for getting a positive result. The protein-rich liquid includes:

- Sugar-free protein shakes

- Thin creamed soup and broth

- Non-fat sugar-free puddings

- Low-carb yogurt

- Split pea or lentil soup

- All food in stage one.

During stage two it recommends you to consume about 3 liters of liquid diet per day. Avoid sugary and carbonated liquids during stage two.

STAGE THREE DIET: PUREE

Stage three begins after two weeks of gastric sleeve surgery. It allows you to include pureed soft food into your diet. The foods like mashed potatoes, fat-free yogurts, thick and smooth soups, baked beans. You are allowed to eat these diets in small quantity about 4 to 5 times daily. Food allowed during stage three is:

- Puree no sugar added fruits

- Tofu

- Pureed peas and lentils

- Eggs

- Plain yogurt

- Steamed or boiled vegetables.

STAGE FOUR DIET: SOLID FOOD

Stage four begins after the four weeks of gastric sleeve surgery. It allows you to take soft solid food in the diet. Try to consume protein-rich foods because it recommends that you should consume at least 60 grams of protein in your daily meal. At this stage, your stomach should be fit to handle solid food. During this stage, you can consume three meals with some snacks. The solid foods allowed in this stage are:

- Lentil and beans soup

- Hot cereals

- Fish

- Boil potatoes

- Soft fruits without skin

- Low-fat cheese

- Lean ground turkey, chicken, beef, pork

- Cooked vegetables.

During this stage, you should avoid whole milk products, snacks, and sugary drinks, fibrous vegetables like broccoli, celery, asparagus, starchy foods like white potatoes, pasta and bread, spicy foods, processed and fried fast food, ETC.

HOW DOES THE GASTRIC SLEEVE WORK?

After gastric sleeve surgery, your stomach is holding a smaller amount of food because during surgery near about 75 to 80 percent of parts of your stomach are removed from your body. It helps you to reduce your food carving and weight loss process.

The surgery also removes the part of the stomach that produces Ghrelin. Ghrelin is one of the gut hormones produced in your stomach, it is also called hunger hormones. Removing these hormones from your body will reduce your hunger feeling and also help to reduce your appetite. By removing these hormones from your stomach, you can easily reduce you're overweight.

ADVANTAGES OF GASTRIC BARIATRIC SLEEVE SURGERY

Gastric Bariatric Sleeve Surgery is an insignificantly obtrusive medical procedure to decrease the size of the stomach. It is currently the most mainstream weight reduction in medical procedures all around the world. People frequently observe the extraordinary achievement that their loved ones have had with the sleeve surgery and, at that point, need similar outcomes. Patients accomplish substantial weight reduction with a straightforward activity without too much stress. It bodes well that with a little stomach, you will be able to eat less and lose a lot of weight. The sleeve surgery has been seen as substantially more potent than the gastric band surgery. It does not require the arrangement of an outside gadget or needle modifications, which the later needs.

Following are some advantages that come alongside this surgery:

Hauling around unreasonable weight puts a great deal of pressure on your joints, regularly causing incessant agony and joint harm. The noteworthy and supported weight reduction that happens after bariatric medical procedures diminishes the weight on joints and regularly permits individuals to quit utilizing torment prescriptions and appreciate considerably more mobility.

Accomplishing and supporting a typical weight territory regularly permits individuals with rest apnea to quit utilizing a CPAP machine at sleep time.

Bariatric medical procedure causes long haul reduction of hard-to-control type 2 diabetes. The aftereffects of this strategy are exceptionally viable for obese or overweight patients with type 2 diabetes, permitting practically all patients to stay liberated from insulin and subordinate prescriptions for about three years post the medical procedure.

Numerous hefty individuals feel discouraged due to helpless self-perception and social shame. Considerably more young individuals who convey a critical abundance of weight think that it is hard to partake in exercises they may somehow appreciate, prompting social separation and discouragement that lead to depression. Losing this weight can enhance enthusiastic well-being in these patients.

Weight reduction medical procedure can likewise improve fertility conditions during childbearing years.

Weight reduction medical procedure can mitigate metabolic disorder, pregnancy entanglements, gallbladder ailment, and that is just the beginning.

With heftiness and its related wellbeing inconveniences increasing at an alarming rate in the world, bariatric medical procedure unquestionably speaks to be an incredible asset for giving supported alleviation to overweight individuals.

Chapter 3

LIFE POST-BARIATRIC SURGERY

PAIN 1 TO 3 MONTHS POST SURGERY

A patient can expect minor pain and swelling for up to three months post-surgery. The pain should be minor but still noticeable, especially when partaking in any sort of physical activity that stretches or contorts the abdomen. This will subside as the weeks go on, and by around the three-month point a patient will no longer need pain medication.

In today's climate, with the increased awareness of the dangers of pain medication, it is doubtful that a doctor would issue a prescription for very long. A patient should follow their doctor's recommendation about what pain medication to take and with what frequency. They shouldn't try and tough it out, but it's important to note that taking medication for a long period of time can cause minor symptoms of withdrawal once the medication is fully removed from a patient's regimen.

An additional note is that for the first week or two that a patient significantly reduces their pain medication; they can expect rapid changes in their bowel movements. A patient will be on medication for a minimum of three weeks, and this long period of time creates a constant state of constipation for the patient. This will subside, but it does so in a fairly rapid way; it's something that should be expected but not something that is all too disruptive to a patient's life.

DIET AFTER 1 MONTH

At around the one month point, a patient will start to consume solid foods again. They must not be overly acidic, and they must be taken with a fair amount of vitamin pills. These are special supplements that are prescribed by a patient's doctor and are a necessity to ensure proper nutrition for a patient. A patient must also continue to drink lots of water; much of the water that was obtained by the patient before the surgery was received through the solid food they were eating. While solid foods are back in the diet, they are consuming far fewer calories and need to supplement this with an increase in liquids.

It is possible that even when a patient is ready to consume solid foods, it will be difficult. This comes from the shrunken stomach, but also from the pain and swelling of the passage leading to the stomach. If solid foods are difficult to eat, a patient should blend them with fat-free milk, water, or broth. For many, broth preserves some of the flavor that is otherwise lost when blending with other liquids and if hot broth is used, it helps to soften the foods even more. It is not suggested that a patient uses a straw to consume these liquids as often the suction causes pain in the esophagus, a result of the swelling from the surgery of the stomach and a slight buildup of acids around the lower section of the throat. For most, at around the two-month point, this additional restriction of no straws can be removed.

Energy levels during this period are still diminished from a lack of calories being taken in, however patients typically experience extra energy from the quick rate of weight loss in these early months. The body is starting to get into a state of ketosis, that is burning fat instead of glucose for energy. This is variable depending on the age of the patient, the physical activity they get post-surgery, as well as the state of their liver. Healthier livers are more efficient at having the body gain energy from ketosis.

DIET AFTER 6 TO 8 MONTHS AND BEYOND

At around six months, a patient will switch to their maintenance diet. This is the beginning of the learning process for how they will eat for the rest of their lives. In addition to the doctors a patient is already familiar with, a nutritionist is also involved. At this stage, it is the nutritionist who actually becomes one of the most important medical professionals for a patient. They will calculate the macros that a patient needs, as well as assist in determining the vitamins and supplements that are needed. Beyond eight months, appointments with a nutritionist will be consistent, but not as frequent as once a month. The macros for a diet typically do not change that much after the eight to nine-month range, and instead it is about ensuring that a patient can maintain their current diet and have enough energy throughout the day. Modifications are made based on the amount of physical activity and energy levels of the patient.

A patient will feel very full, so there are very small amounts of food. This is because of the shrunken stomach, but also because some degree of swelling still exists. This is a great time to develop new habits, typically behavior that is the opposite of what caused a patient to need bariatric surgery in the first place. Eating slowly and savoring every bite is a key component of these new eating habits. Typically a patient would have eaten much faster leading up to surgery, rarely savoring the taste of food and instead going for volume. Trying to keep this habit going post-surgery is a recipe for extreme stomach pain as more food can be ingested before it is sensed by the body that it simply cannot contain that much volume.

This is a great time to also start learning how to cook and become more intimate with food. Part of the issue with eating disorders is that abstinence is not a solution like it is for other behavioral addictions. A healthy relationship must be maintained with food, as it is something that cannot be cut out completely. In addition, when and with whom a patient eats is a factor in their success. Eating should be an activity to itself and should not be done on the run or in front of a computer or television. Good eating habits start with eating at the same time each day and using it as a time for the family to discuss their day.

WEIGHT LOSS IN THE LONG TERM – PLATEAUS AND AVOIDING OLD HABITS

The weight loss that a patient experiences is a reason for joy, but after the two-year point there will be a plateau. This is not inherently a bad thing, and the patient is still going to be losing weight, albeit at a far slower rate. The issue is it can be difficult for a patient to adapt to the mental challenges of this slower rate of change. Bariatric surgery is a tool to assist in weight loss but it's not a solution by itself.

A patient must be willing to make long-term changes in their relationship with food and how they incorporate exercise into their life. It will be impossible for a patient to go back to their old weight, but it is quite possible to have a patient revert to their old mindset. Sticking to a diet, changing one's relationship with food, and adding exercise to their routine is the only surefire way to avoid old habits that led to bariatric surgery and the poor mental state associated with it.

Chapter 4

LIFE POST-BARIATRIC SURGERY

STAGE ONE

Food and Drink Choices

You need to follow your doctor's orders as far as when, how much, and what foods you can consume after your gastric sleeve surgery. However, this guide can give you an idea of what to expect.

Surgery day - The staff will put you on intravenous fluid, but you will have to drink about one fluid ounce of water (and only water) per hour. You will be given one-ounce medicine cups to measure out and sip your water from, and you will be required to make notes regarding your water intake.

Day One - Usually by noon on the day following your surgery, you will start to consume between one and three ounces of broth, sugar-free gelatin, decarbonized ("flat") diet ginger ale, or water per hour.

You will need to stop drinking as soon as you feel full. Don't force yourself to drink more than you are comfortable drinking. However, the goal will be for you to reach a drinking capacity of one quart (32 ounces) per day. You will likely reach that goal within that day. Once you do, the intravenous fluids can be discontinued.

Day Two - Usually by the second day out from your surgery, you will take in low-sugar, enriched liquids. You will do this for two to three weeks.

You will take in four fluid ounces of a nutritional supplement every other hour over an eight-hour period per day. Between these supplements, you will drink between four and eight fluid ounces of various clear liquids.

These liquids include the following:

- Decaffeinated herbal tea

- Decaffeinated coffee

- Fruit juice (no added sugar, max 4 ounces per serving and 8 ounces daily)

- Sugar-free popsicles (under 20 calories, up to two daily)

- Tomato juice

- V-8 juice

- Flat diet decaffeinated soda

- Broth

- Sugar-free drinks like kool-aid or crystal light

- Water.

Fluid goal: The fluid goal is for you to reach a capacity of six cups of liquid per day of both the nutrient-enriched beverage and the clear liquids. Stop when full, though, and don't push things beyond what is comfortable.

Protein goal: You will need to consume at least 70 grams of protein per day, which is usually what is in seven scoops of protein powder. You will need to track your protein intake.

Supplements: Take these with your meals. You will need to take two multivitamins in chewable form in addition to three 600 mg of calcium carbonate and vitamin D in chewable form daily.

Reminders: Take 30 minutes to sip your liquids and continue to record all food and fluid intake.

The Clear Liquids Diet

A clear liquid diet is recommended in the post-op stage after the gastric sleeve surgery. It is mainly because that few days after the surgery, the healing phase initiates, and the stomach isn't capable of processing nutrients and calories in the food, but the body does need hydration. Clear liquid provides much-needed minerals, metabolites, and moisture that the body needs; therefore, they are given to a person after the surgery for a quick recovery. The following are the clear liquids that must be consumed on the bariatric diet.

- Broth

- Unsweetened juice

- Decaffeinated tea or coffee

- Milk (skim or 1 percent)

- Sugar-free gelatine drinks.

The rule of thumb for clear liquids is that it's either you can see through the glass—side to side or the water is thin enough that it's flowing freely, and you can somehow see through from side to side.

You are to consume only light liquids for the following 2 to 3 days or after your admission from the hospital.

Examples of clear liquids you can consume after the surgery include:

Tap water

Pure fruit juices – refrain from drinking commercially processed or powdered juices.

Broths or soups– vegetables, beef, or chicken are okay, but make sure that it's clear and no solid sediments are present.

Other clear liquids may include decaffeinated coffee or tea and calorie-free sports drink.

Important notes before you delve into these recipes:

Keeping yourself hydrated is the most crucial part a few days after your surgery. You should drink 48 to 64 ounces or 6 to 8 glass of water per day.

Never serve recipes either cold or hot for around 6 weeks until you have fully recovered from the surgery. Consuming extreme foods might cause gastric problems and compromise surgical procedure.

When consuming fruit juices, make sure that they are fresh and natural. Also, dilute them thoroughly to obtain a steady liquid consistency and strain them to remove excess solid compounds. This process is to avoid the development of diarrhea or nausea.

However, you have to bear in mind that your stomach is still recovering after surgery. Thus, you may still experience episodes of nausea or vomiting, but these are common, and you have nothing to worry about. Again, we emphasize that you always hydrate yourself to alleviate the above symptoms.

Also, it has to be noted that food choices during this phase are limited. Thus, the recipes presented below are easy and simple to make, which mainly revolves around broths and juices.

Also, you don't really have to concern yourself with what to prepare because the hospital got you covered. They will provide the necessary clear liquids to aid your recovery process.

But if you want to add a personal touch to your meals, then the following recipes are guaranteed delicious and, most importantly, nutritious and aid recovery.

Pure Fruit Juices: Important reminder: since solid compounds are not allowed for a few days after surgery, you have to take extra precautionary steps. While blenders liquefy solid foods, some solid compounds may still peak through. Thus, we recommend you to use strainers in each of the juice recipes to remove solid compounds.

GOOD CHOICES OF CLEAR FLUIDS

1. Water.

2. Tea – warm traditional, fruit or herbal teas.

3. Coffee – warm, ideally decaffeinated.

4. 'No-added-sugar' or 'sugar-free' squashes and cordials.

5. Bovril, marmite or oxo 'salty' drinks diluted well with hot water.

6. Sugar-free ice lollies.

7. Sugar-free jelly, made up as per packet instructions.

8. Chicken, beef or vegetable bouillon/broth/consommé or clear soup.

9. A whey protein isolate fruit drink like syntrax nectar, made up with water –great for getting protein in the early days.

1. GREEN GIANT JUICE

5 min

0 min

Liquids Diet

2 Servings

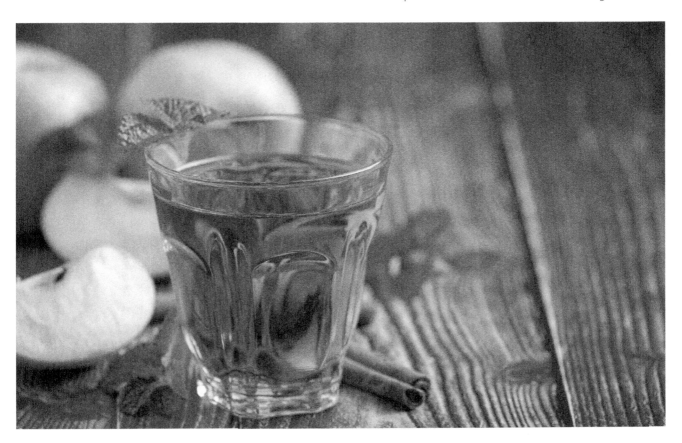

INGREDIENTS

- 1 medium-sized apple, cored
- 1 large-sized cucumber
- 3 to 6 small sized celery, remove the end of the stalks
- Water (optional).

DIRECTIONS

1. Juice all the ingredients in the order listed according to the manufacturer's instructions.

2. Serve immediately.

3. If the taste is strong for you, you may add some water depending on your preference.

NUTRITION (per serving): Calories: 83 kcal | Fats: 0g | Carbs: 9g | Protein: 1g.

2. ASIAN PEAR/BEET JUICE

5 min

0 min

Liquids Diet

2 Servings

INGREDIENTS

- 1 Asian pear
- 1 apple
- 1 beet
- 1 carrot
- ½ cup cabbage
- 3 handfuls chard.

DIRECTIONS

1. Juice all the ingredients in the order listed according to the manufacturer's instructions.
2. Serve immediately.

NUTRITION (per serving): Calories: 123 kcal | Fats: 0g | Carbs: 19g | Protein: 1g.

3. FRESH GREEN JUICE

5 min

0 min

Liquids Diet

2 Servings

INGREDIENTS

- 5-6 kale leaves
- 1 cucumber
- 3-4 celery stalks
- 2 apples
- ½ lemon, peeled or sliced.

DIRECTIONS

1. Juice all the ingredients in the order listed according to the manufacturer's instructions.
2. Serve immediately.

NUTRITION (per serving): Calories: 53 kcal | Fats: 0g | Carbs: 13g | Protein: 1g.

4. CARROT PINEAPPLE ORANGE JUICE

5 min

0 min

Liquids Diet

2 Servings

INGREDIENTS

- 1 small orange, including rind, seeded and cut into pieces
- ⅛ small, ripe pineapple, peeled, cored and cut into pieces
- 2 carrots, scrubbed clean and cut into pieces
- ½ lemon Juice, stirred in at end.

DIRECTIONS

1. Juice all the ingredients in the order listed according to the manufacturer's instructions.
2. Serve immediately.

NUTRITION (per serving): Calories: 113 kcal | Fats: 0g | Carbs: 9g | Protein: 0g.

5. DETOX JUICE

5 min

0 min

Liquids Diet

2 Servings

INGREDIENTS

- 1 Asian pear
- 1 apple
- 1 beet
- 1 carrot
- ½ cup cabbage
- 3 handfuls chard.

DIRECTIONS

1. Juice all the ingredients in the order listed according to the manufacturer's instructions.
2. Serve immediately.

NUTRITION (per serving): Calories: 126 kcal | Fats: 0g | Carbs: 13g | Protein: 1g.

6. RICH ANTIOXIDANT JUICE

5 min

0 min

Liquids Diet

2 Servings

INGREDIENTS

- 3 medium carrots, peeled
- 2 medium beets, cleaned and brushed
- 1 Green apple such as Granny Smith, peeled and cored.

DIRECTIONS

1. Juice all the ingredients in the order listed according to the manufacturer's instructions.
2. Serve immediately.

NUTRITION (per serving): Calories: 123 kcal | Fats: 0g | Carbs: 19g | Protein: 1g.

7. BLOOD ORANGE SPORTS DRINK

5 min

0 min

Liquids Diet

2 Servings

INGREDIENTS

- 2 cups of coconut water
- 1 medium blood orange, squeezed
- 1½ tbsp. of honey or 1 packet of Stevia sugar
- Pinch of salt.

DIRECTIONS

1. Combine all ingredients together, and mix well.
2. Serve immediately.

NUTRITION (per serving): Calories: 234 kcal | Fats: 4g | Carbs: 27g | Protein: 2g.

8. LIME & MINT INFUSION

 5 min 0 min Liquids Diet 2 Servings

INGREDIENTS

- 2 cups of cold water
- 1 large lime, sliced
- ½ cup of lightly packed spearmint leaves
- 1 package of Stevia sugar.

DIRECTIONS

1. In a 1-quart glass container or larger, lightly mash the lime and spearmint leaves with the pestle.
2. Add iced cold water. Stir well.
3. Optional: add Stevia to taste.

NUTRITION (per serving): Calories: 75 kcal | Fats: 0g | Carbs: 23g | Protein: 0g.

9. STRAWBERRY ICED TEA

 5 min 0 min Liquids Diet 2 Servings

INGREDIENTS

- 6-10 medium strawberries, chopped
- 1 tsp. lemon juice
- 2 cups of brewed white tea, chilled
- ½ - 1 tsp. honey or Stevia sugar (optional).

DIRECTIONS

1. Puree the strawberries until smooth consistency. Then strain through fine cheesecloth on top of a metal strainer to remove the seeds.
2. Combine the strained strawberry mixture with lemon juice and white tea.
3. Mix well. Add honey or Stevia to taste.

NUTRITION (per serving): Calories: 127 kcal | Fats: 0g | Carbs: 24g | Protein: 1g.

10. WATERMELON POPSICLES

 5 min

 0 min

 Liquids Diet

 2 Servings

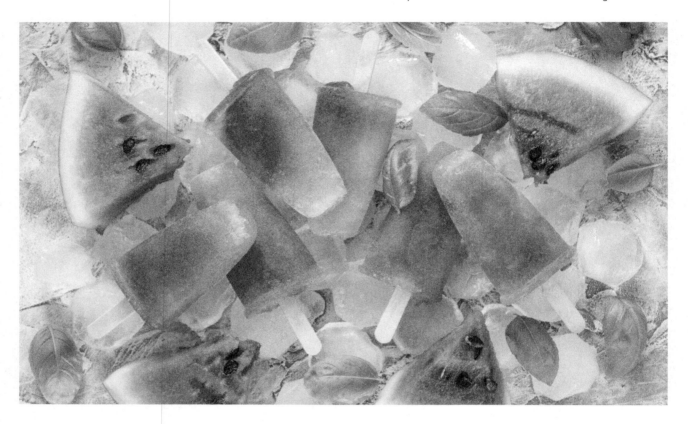

INGREDIENTS

- 2 cups watermelon juice (no sugar added store bought juice or homemade freshly pressed juice)
- ½ tbsp. lime juice
- 1 tsp. honey or Stevia sugar (optional).

DIRECTIONS

1. Mix all ingredients together.
2. Carefully transfer mixture to the mold of your choice.
3. Freeze overnight.

NUTRITION (per serving): Calories: 135 kcal | Fats: 0g | Carbs: 22g | Protein: 1g.

11. HOMEMADE CHICKEN BROTH

15 min

2 h 30 min

Liquids Diet

6 Servings

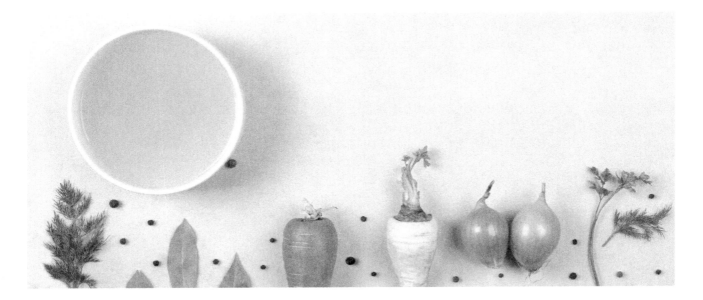

INGREDIENTS

- 2 lbs. bone-in skin on chicken
- 2 large carrots, cleaned and thick sliced
- 2 medium onions, quartered
- 3 celery sticks with leaves, cut into chunks
- 8 whole peppercorns
- 1 tsp. thyme, dried
- 1 tsp. rosemary, dried
- 2 cups of water
- Salt to taste.

DIRECTIONS

1. Combine everything in a pot except the salt. Bring to a boil.
2. Skim the floating foam.
3. Lower the heat. Simmer for about 2 hours until the meat can be easily removed from the bone.
4. Strain vegetables, bones, meats, and spices from the broth and discard the solids.
5. Season broth with salt to taste.
6. Let the broth cool or refrigerate overnight. Skim the fat for a leaner broth.

NUTRITION (per serving): Calories: 75 kcal | Fats: 0g | Carbs: 23g | Protein: 0g.

12. GINGER CHICKEN SOUP

15 min   2 h 30 min   Liquids Diet   6 Servings

Healthy and lean homemade chicken soup with garlic, ginger, and lemongrass. The aromatic lemongrass add freshness to the broth with a hint of spiciness from the ginger. The best to enjoy this broth warm.

This homemade chicken stock can be refrigerated for 2 days or frozen for 1 month to prolong shelf life.

INGREDIENTS

- 6-10 medium strawberries, chopped
- 1 tsp. lemon juice
- 2 cups of brewed white tea, chilled
- ½ - 1 tsp. honey or Stevia sugar (optional).

DIRECTIONS

1. Puree the strawberries until smooth consistency. Then strain through fine cheesecloth on top of a metal strainer to remove the seeds.

2. Combine the strained strawberry mixture with lemon juice and white tea.

3. Mix well. Add honey or Stevia to taste.

NUTRITION (per serving): Calories: 127 kcal | Fats: 0g | Carbs: 24g | Protein: 1g.

Chapter 5

POST OPERATION
SOFT & PUREED FOODS

STAGE TWO

Two to Three Weeks Out – Two or three weeks after your surgery, you can gradually introduce pureed and soft food that resembles the consistency of applesauce and up to a very soft consistency.

You will consume thick liquids, such as protein shakes and pureed food, using your blender for most of what you consume during this phase. Because of their high protein content, the protein shakes will be useful to you on days when you are having trouble reaching your daily intake of protein.

You won't be using a straw (because it might introduce air to your stomach), but the food will need to be blended so small that it could fit through a straw.

Your pureed food will resemble baby food. In fact, you can eat baby food, but only the pureed meat ones contain the protein you need. You will probably enjoy pureed meat that you make yourself better, though.

You may not be able to tolerate meat until later on in this stage. You can see how you do with meat later on if you want to. There are many other tasty choices available that will give you the protein and other nutrients you need.

You need to have six meals per day and take the supplements and liquids in between meal times, not with the meals. Remember to chew well all food that needs to be chewed.

SOFT/PUREED FOOD COOKING TIPS AND MENU IDEAS FOR YOUR STAGE TWO DIET

You'll want to ease into this stage by consuming things like Lactaid-free milk, almond milk, unsweetened coconut milk, blended Greek yogurt with no fruit chunks, unsweetened applesauce, cooked cereal such as oatmeal, grits, or Cream of Wheat made with lactose-free milk, blended soup made with lactose-free milk, blended fruit smoothies, and shakes.

Do not combine food selections below right at first in any one meal, but gradually try the following foods during this phase:

- Light white fish

- Crackers with peanut butter

- Cooked eggs

- Cooked vegetables

- Soft fruit

- Yogurt with fruit

- Cottage cheese

- Oatmeal, grits, or Cream of Wheat

- Blended soup.

You may tolerate meat, however, so you can test your tolerance and see. After all, you won't want to only consume breakfast food and sweet-tasting shakes for longer than you have to.

Below, you can find sources of protein and also food from the various food groups that you ought to begin to consume during this phase.

PROTEIN SOURCES

Protein is essential for our bodies to function properly, and you need to concentrate on consuming liquid protein when you first get out of your surgery. Protein will speed up the healing process, enhance your fat-burning metabolism, and minimize your hair loss.

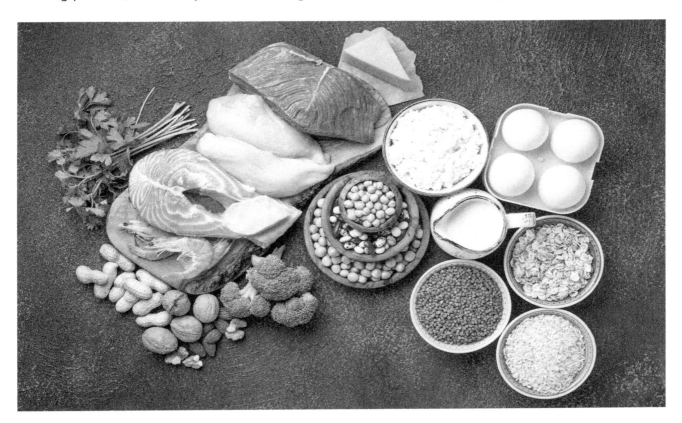

Besides a deficiency in protein, hair loss is also associated with a deficiency in iron and zinc, so you'll need to make sure you take multivitamins. You will probably lose some hair anyway about a half year after your surgery for a little bit, so you will want to be sure that you give it all of the nutrients that you can to eventually come out of this experience thin, with muscle tone and a full head of hair.

Eat lots of protein and take your vitamins! You'll need to take in around 70 grams of protein per day during this phase.

Remember that you will need to mash or puree foods that are not already soft. Here are some good sources of protein:

PROTEIN SOURCE	Serving Size	Gr. Per Serving
Protein powders (for smoothies)	1 scoop	20-40
Cooked vegetables	.5 cup	1-2
Instant breakfast drinks	1 packet	4-15
Tofu	3 oz.	11
Soy veggie burger	1	9
Bread	1 slice	2
Rice	.5 cup	5
Noodles/macaroni	.5 cup	3-4
Dry cereal	1 oz.	5
Oatmeal	1 cup	5
Nuts	.25 cup	4.5
Lima beans	.5 cup	5
Peanut butter	2 tbsp.	8.5
Beans: brown, kidney, black-eyed peas garbanzo, white, pinto, black	.5 cup	7.5
Fat-free refried beans	.5 cup	8
Reduced-fat ricotta cheese	1 oz.	6
Low-fat yogurt	1 cup	8-12
Non-fat milk powder	1 tbsp.	2.5
Skim milk/1% milk	1 cup	8
Low-fat cottage cheese	.5 cup	13
Egg substitute	.25 cup	6
Egg whites	2 tbsp.	9
Egg	1 med	7
Lean meat: pork, beef, fish, chicken	1 oz.	7

Other sources of protein include:

- Nonfat dry milk powder (Add this to hot cereals, soups, casseroles, etc.)

- Legumes

- Fish

- Cream of Wheat with skim milk

- Strained cream soups, such as chicken, mushroom, potato, or celery

- Baby food meats

- White fish, such as orange roughy, tilapia, haddock, and cod

- Canned chicken breast

- Canned tuna in water.

Grains and Starches

You will need to mash or puree foods that are not already soft. Good sources of grains and starches include the following:

- Winter squash

- Mashed potatoes

- Sweet potatoes

- Baby oatmeal

- Grits

- Farina.

Fruit

You will need to mash or puree foods that are not already soft. Good sources of fruit include the following:

- Peaches

- Apricots

- Melons

- Pineapples

- Pears

- Bananas

- Canned fruit in own juices

- Applesauce

- Juice sweetened with a non-nutritive sweetener

- Diluted 100% apple juice

- Diluted 100% grape juice

- Diluted 100% cranberry juice.

Vegetables

You will need to mash or puree foods that are not already soft. Good sources of vegetables include the following:

- Diet V-8 Splash

- V-8 Juice

- Other tomato juice

- Spinach

- Green beans

- Summer squash

- Carrots.

Note: Avoid cauliflower, broccoli, or other fibrous veggies during your stage two, pureed food time.

Drinks

Make sure that you consume at least eight cups of low-calorie, caffeine-free liquids throughout the day so that you will prevent yourself from becoming dehydrated. Sip these drinks between the meals. Do not drink with meals. Wait for 30 to 45 minutes after you finish your meal before you drink fluids. The following items are examples of drinks you can have:

- Sugar-free flavored drinks

- Skim milk

- Decaffeinated coffee (maximum 8 ounces per day)

- Decaffeinated tea (maximum 8 ounces per day)

- Diet fruit drinks (under 10 calories per day)

- Water

- Sugar-free flavored water

- Zero-calorie flavored water.

Supplements

You will also need to start taking supplements daily that contain the following:

- Iron

- Zinc

- Calcium citrate

- B12

- Other supplements as indicated from your lab results.

Take them in chewable form for the first month (something like Flintstones) twice daily. You can start taking vitamins and minerals in pill form after your first post-operative month if you prefer pills.

LACTOSE AND FOOD INTOLERANCES

Some gastric sleeve patients become intolerant to lactose after their surgery, so you'll need to use unsweetened coconut milk, almond milk, or Lactaid-free milk. If you have pain or vomit after you introduce a new kind of food, go back to your liquid diet for an entire day before trying pureed food again. Don't let it discourage you. Notate when you ate the problem food, what food it was that gave you the problem, and what your reaction was to it.

You may not be able to tolerate poultry or other meat for a while after your surgery. If you have trouble tolerating some of the pureed meat, you might want to wait until later in this phase to try meat. You can just label it and freeze it.

Alternatively, you can introduce meat in small amounts, blended in with potatoes or other vegetables and/or sauces. There are recipes for meat dishes in this book that you can make. Many of them are various veggie-rich meatball and sauce meals that you eat in blended form while you are in the early stages after your gastric sleeve surgery.

Food to Avoid

Sugar and carbs can easily sabotage your weight loss efforts, as can bad fats or even good fats if eaten excess. Avoid the following foods to prevent sabotaging your weight loss efforts:

- Fried food

- Doughnuts

- Alcohol

- Ice cream

- Sherbet

- Preserves

- Cakes

- Molasses

- Flavored drink mix

- Honey

- Regular sodas

- Sweets

- Candy.

TIPS FOR THE FIRST MONTH AFTER YOUR OPERATION

Keep food records. You may want to do this indefinitely, just to stay on top of what you're eating, but be sure to do it for that first after your surgery. Notate the following:

- Time you ate

- Type of food you ate

- Amount of food you ate

- How you prepared your food, including any oils used

- Protein gram amount wherever you can find this information.

Use ice trays to control portion size, noting that each cube holds about two ounces. These are good for use with pureed meats and vegetables, low-fat cream soups, etc.

Eat only two to four ounces of food per meal, concentrating on protein intake. Try to get 80 grams of protein daily, which protein shakes and supplements would help you to achieve in addition to what you can eat.

Try to eat between four and six small meals daily.

Take your time eating and drinking. Take half an hour to eat and drink just four ounces, which is half a cup.

Drink at least eight cups of liquids daily between the meals, waiting 30 to 45 minutes after your last meal to drink.

LOW-FAT COOKING TIPS

When you get to where you can eat more solid food, prepare the food items as normal and then just puree/blend or mash them. See how you like the taste. If you don't tolerate meat by itself, you may tolerate a little of it if it is mixed with mashed potatoes, along with low-fat sour cream, or eaten in blended recipe form (See the blended meat recipes).

Poultry and Other Meat

- Use lean meat.

- Top round beef (It's best to forego red meat, however)

- Turkey, no skin, white meat

- Chicken, no skin, white meat

- Trim off the fat

- Use low-fat cooking methods

- Broil, grill, bake, sauté, stir-fry using broth, vegetable spray, a small amount of oil, or water

- Drain off fat.

Vegetables

- Use "I Can't Believe It's Not Butter" spray for butter flavor without the calories.

- Add tomatoes, carrots, green peppers, and other fresh vegetables to your spaghetti sauces.

- Add fat-free sour cream or low-fat cottage cheese to potatoes.

- Cook using methods that do not require fat, such as microwave, steam, grill, and bake.

- Don't cook with bacon, butter, or fatback.

- Avoid high-fat sauces, such as butter, oil, cheese, and sauces made with cream.

Soups

- Let your soup cool. Skim fat off after it has cooled, accumulated on the top, and hardened.

Desserts

- Use Splenda to add sweetness to smoothies, shakes, unsweetened decaffeinated tea, etc.

- Read food labels. Only consider food items that have low sugar content or use artificial sweeteners.

Soft Foods

When you transitioned to phase 3 of your recovery process, you can now move on to more solid foods, which include whole-wheat cereals, fish, chicken, vegetables, and fresh fruits.

Things to keep in mind after the first month of recovery:

1. Chew your food thoroughly before swallowing.

2. Continue to drink your 6 to 8 cups of water.

3. Intake of high-protein foods or supplements. Consume them before meals. The General recommended intake is 50 to 60 grams of protein for women and 60 to 70 grams for men.

4. In consuming dietary supplements, choose those that are chewable.

5. Refrain from eating foods that contain high levels of calories.

6. Do not drink while you're eating. Doing so can cause your stomach to fill quickly.

7. Drink liquids 30 minutes after you've finished your meal.

8. Because you'll be restricting calorie intake, it's essential that you take dietary supplements regularly.

GOOD CHOICES OF FULL LIQUIDS

1. Milk – skimmed, semi-skimmed, almond, soya, oat, rice and Flora Proactive.

2. Milky chai type tea – lightly-spiced for added flavors.

3. Yogurt without added sugar and fruit bits.

4. Whey protein isolate drinks, icy, cold or warm made up with milk or water.

5. Ice cream made with whey protein isolate powder mixed with milk or water.

6. Mashed potato mixed with a little broth or gravy until thin and soup-like.

7. Fresh homemade fruit juice without added sugar and diluted with water.

8. V8 or tomato juice – warm or chilled.

9. Home-made, not too thick smoothies diluted if necessary, with water.

10. Simple home-made cocoa (made with 2 tablespoons unsweetened cocoa powder and 1 cup semi-skimmed milk).

11. Unsweetened and low-fat hot chocolate drinks.

12. Smooth cream-style low-fat soups.

13. Home-made vegetable, fish or poultry soups, pureed until smooth and diluted to a smooth runny consistency (gradually increase the thickness as you progress through this stage to the next soft or pureed food stage).

14. Very gently set egg custards.

15. Low-sugar and low-fat custards.

GOOD CHOICES OF SOFT FOODS

1. Porridge, oat with semi-skimmed milk and runny consistency.

2. Mashed banana with a little yogurt if liked or with a low-fat and low-sugar custard.

3. Scrambled eggs cooked very soft.

4. Very soft and gently cooked plain omelet.

5. A soft-boiled egg or poached one.

6. Plain low-fat cottage cheese.

7. Low-sugar and low-fat fromage frais.

8. Pureed chicken or turkey in gravy.

9. Pureed fish (salmon, tuna, pilchards or mackerel) in a thin tomato sauce.

10. Soft and smooth low-fat pate or spread.

11. Pureed boiled vegetables such as potato, pumpkin, cauliflower or carrot with thin gravy or mixed with grated low-fat cheese or low-fat cream cheese.

12. Pureed casserole and stew dishes of a thinnish consistency.

13. Pureed, thickened or soft piece vegetable and chicken soups.

14. Smooth and light low-sugar and low-fat milk mousse.

15. Milky pudding such as tapioca, sago or rice but keep sugar to a minimum.

16. Soft lentils, beans and peas, mashed or pureed for a little texture.

17. Silken or smooth tofu.

18. Thick fruit and vegetable smoothies.

19. Pureed avocado.

20. Low-sugar sorbets.

13. GREEN BOOSTER SMOOTHIE

 5 min

 0 min

 Soft &Pureed food

 2 Servings

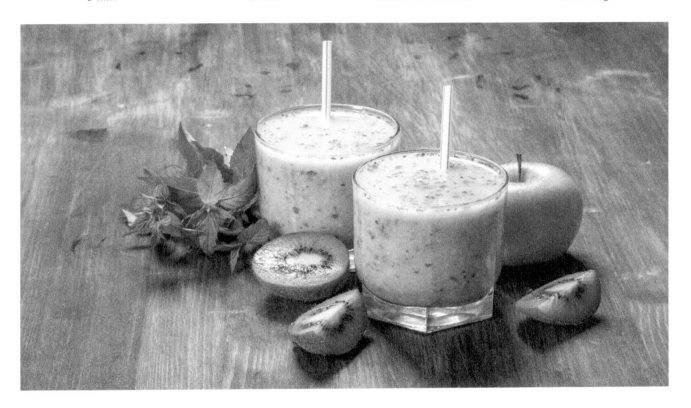

INGREDIENTS

- 1 cup of mango, peeled and cubes
- 1 head of baby romaine lettuce (or spinach), chopped
- 1 kiwi fruit, peeled and diced
- 1 cucumber, peeled and diced
- 1 medium-sized apple, cored.

DIRECTIONS

1. Blend mango, lettuce and kiwi.
2. Juice apple and cucumber.
3. Next, blend all together.
4. If the taste is strong for you, you may add some water or ice, depending on your preference.

NUTRITION (per serving): Calories: 253 kcal | Fats: 4g | Carbs: 39g | Protein: 18g.

14. STRAWBERRY-APPLE JUICE DELIGHT

5 min

0 min

Soft & Pureed food

2 Servings

INGREDIENTS

- 1 medium-sized apple, peeled and cored
- 2 cups of strawberries with their tops removed.

DIRECTIONS

1. Juice or blend the strawberries first.
2. Last, blend or juice the apples and mix them with the strawberry juice.

NUTRITION (per serving): Calories: 120 kcal | Fat: 0g | Carbs: 30g | Protein: 0g.

15. IMMUNE BOOSTERS

5 min

0 min

Soft & Pureed food

2 Servings

INGREDIENTS

- 1 cup of blueberries
- 2 medium-sized raw beets, cut into quarters
- 1 cup of strawberries, with top ends removed.

DIRECTIONS

1. First, put all the ingredients in a blender.
2. Then blend them until the mixture becomes liquid.

NUTRITION (per serving): Calories: 10 kcal | Fats: 0g | Carbs: 4g | Protein: 0g.

16. TROPICAL GREEN PARADISE

 5 min 0 min Soft & Pureed food 2 Servings

INGREDIENTS

- 1 medium-sized cucumber
- 8 to 10 pieces of celery stalks
- 1 small-sized honeydew.

DIRECTIONS

1. Put all the ingredients together in a blender.
2. Then blend them until a liquid consistency is achieved.

NUTRITION (per serving): Calories: 15 kcal | Fats: 0g | Carbs: 6g | Protein: 0g.

17. BEET & BERRY DELUXE

 5 min 0 min Soft & Pureed food 2 Servings

INGREDIENTS

- ⅓ cup of raw beets, peeled and chopped
- 1⅓ cup of fresh strawberries
- ⅔ cup of pure apple juice
- ¼ ripe bananas (optional).

DIRECTIONS

1. Mix all the ingredients in a blender and blend them until a smooth and creamy texture is obtained.
2. Adjust flavor based on your preference: add strawberries for more fruity taste, bananas for sweetness, or apple juice to make the texture thinner.

NUTRITION (per serving): Calories: 40 kcal | Fats: 2g | Carbs: 3g | Protein: 20g.

18. AFTERNOON SUNSHINE

5 min

0 min

Soft & Pureed food

2 Servings

A serving of afternoon sunshine is sure to boost your energy during your admission.

INGREDIENTS

- 1 ripe banana, chopped
- 6 cubes fat-free soy milk
- 6 cubes of fat-free skim milk.

DIRECTIONS

1. Put all the ingredients together in a blender.
2. Then blend them until a liquid consistency is achieved.

NUTRITION (per serving): Calories: 80 kcal | Fats: 1g | Carbs: 17g | Protein: 0g.

19. PINK REFRESHER

10 min

0 min

Soft & Pureed food

2 Servings

INGREDIENTS

- 2 cups of watermelon
- 1 cup of cucumber
- 1 cup of water.

DIRECTIONS

1. Add water, cucumber, and watermelon in a blender.
2. Mix them until a smooth and liquid consistency is achieved.

NUTRITION (per serving): Calories: 140 kcal | Fats: 2.5g | Carbs: 27g | Protein: 1g.

20. APPLE BANANA SMOOTHIE

10 min

0 min

Soft & Pureed food

1 Servings

INGREDIENTS

- ½ cup no-sugar apple juice
- ½ banana, peeled and sliced
- ½ cup skim milk
- 5 ice cubes
- Stevia sugar, to taste.

DIRECTIONS

1. Put all the ingredients together in a blender.
2. Then blend them until smooth.

NUTRITION (per serving): Calories: 80 kcal | Fats: 1g | Carbs: 17g | Protein: 0g.

21. PEANUT & BANANA PROTEIN SHAKE

5 min

0 min

Soft & Pureed food

1 Servings

INGREDIENTS

- 1 scoop chocolate flavored whey protein
- ½ banana, peeled and cut
- 1-2 tbsp. peanut butter
- ½ cup ice cubes
- ½ cup water or non-fat milk.

DIRECTIONS

1. Put all the ingredients together in a blender.
2. Then blend them until smooth.

NUTRITION (per serving): Calories: 113 kcal | Fats: 7g | Carbs: 21g | Protein: 19g.

22. CREAMY ZUCCHINI SOUP

15 min

16 min

Soft & Pureed food

4 Servings

A simple, creamy, sublimely silky zucchini soup.

This low fat/calorie soup is tasty and healthy.

INGREDIENTS

- 1 tbsp. coconut oil
- 1 medium yellow onion
- 3 garlic cloves
- 4 zucchinis
- 2 turnips
- ¼ cup fresh cilantro
- 2 tbsp. chopped fresh mint
- 2 tsp. curry powder
- ½ tsp. cumin powder
- 2 cups vegetable broth
- Salt and black pepper, to taste
- 1¼ cups almond milk
- 1 tbsp. plain vinegar
- ¼ tsp. red chili flakes.

DIRECTIONS

1. Warm up coconut oil in a big pot and sauté the onion for 3 minutes or until softened.

2. Stir in the garlic and cook for 30 seconds or until fragrant.

3. Mix in the zucchinis, turnips, cilantro, mint, curry powder, cumin powder, and vegetable broth. Season with salt, black pepper, and stir well.

4. Boil then, simmer for 10 minutes.

5. With an immersion blender to puree the ingredients until smooth.

6. Stir in the almond milk, vinegar, and simmer for 2 minutes.

7. Serve warm.

NUTRITION (per serving): Calories: 160 kcal | Fats: 10g | Carbs: 3.4g | Protein: 7.5g.

23. CREAMY CORN DELIGHT

| 10 min | 5 min | Soft & Pureed food | 4 Servings |

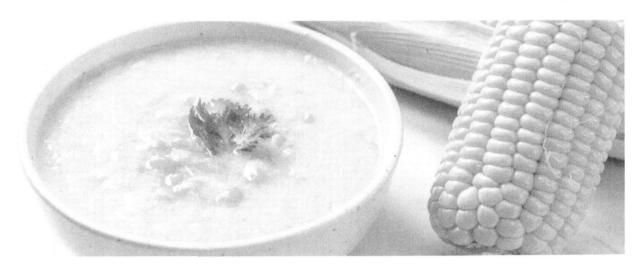

INGREDIENTS

- 3 cups whole kernel corn, canned or boiled
- ½ tbsp. cornstarch
- 3 tbsp. cream of corn powder
- ½ cup evaporated milk
- 1 tbsp. vegetable oil
- 2 eggs, beaten
- Salt, to taste
- Ground pepper, to taste
- 4 cups water.

DIRECTIONS

1. Dissolve cream of corn and cornstarch in a half cup of water. Set them aside for a moment.
2. Place the remaining 3½ of water in a cooking pot and heat over medium-high temperature.
3. Next, add all the remaining ingredients to the cooking pot.
4. Stir until all the ingredients dissolve.
5. Pour in the mixture of cream corn and cornstarch.
6. Heat the cooking pot until it boils.
7. Reduce the temperature and allow it to simmer for 1 to 2 minutes while continually stirring.
8. If you desire a much thinner soup, then add water. Adjust to personal preference, accordingly.

NUTRITION (per serving): Calories: 107 kcal | Fats: 10g | Carbs: 2g | Protein: 8g.

24. CREAMY TOMATO SOUP DELUXE WITH NAVY BEANS

6 h 15 min

2 h

Soft & Pureed food

4 Servings

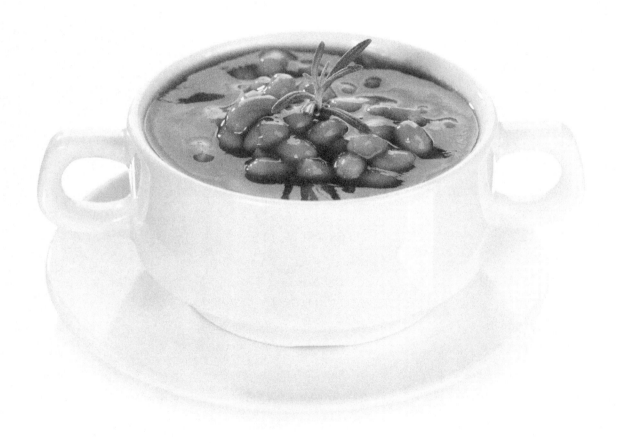

INGREDIENTS

- 1 small can tomato paste
- 1 can tomatoes
- 1 cup navy beans

DIRECTIONS

1. First is to soften the beans by soaking them in cold water for 6 hours.

2. After the beans have softened, drain and rinse the beans. Replace it with another set of cold water that's 3 times more

- 4 cups vegetable broth
- 2 tbsp. olive oil
- 3 medium-sized carrots, peeled and then finely chopped
- 1 large-sized leek, chopped thinly
- 1 tbsp. salt
- 2 to 4 cloves garlic, thinly sliced
- 3 tbsp. raw honey
- 2 cups kale, finely chopped
- 1 tbsp. dried dill.

than the first batch of water.

3. Place the beans in a large cooking pot and boil over medium-high heat.

4. Once it reached boiling point, turn the heat down by a notch and allow it to simmer. Cooking the beans may take up to 90 minutes.

5. After the beans are tenderized, drain the water and rinse the beans with cold water. Set them aside for a moment.

6. Place olive oil in cooking oil and heat over medium-high heat. Add in carrots and leeks and pour in 1 tablespoon of salt. And then cook it for roughly 5 to 8 minutes, or until the leeks dehydrate.

7. Add the garlic and cook for another 2 to 3 minutes until it provides a strong fragrance.

8. Next is to add vegetable broth, tomato paste, tomatoes, and dill. Stir them together until the mixture is thoroughly diluted.

9. Again, turn the heat up a notch to induce a gentle boil.

10. Once it boiled, turn it down again to a simmer. Cook for about 15 minutes until the vegetables are tender.

11. Now, add kale, honey, and the beans we cooked earlier. Stir the mixture thoroughly.

12. Cook for 3 to 4 minutes until kale is soft.

13. Transfer 2/3 of the mixture in a separate bowl and use an immersion blender. Blend until a smooth and liquid consistency is attained.

14. Add the unblended 1/3 part of the mixture into the blended one. When mixed properly, it will present a creamy and silky texture.

15. Put the cooking pot back in the heat. Heat them for a few minutes to allow the flavors to sync.

16. Garnish it with tiny amounts of peanut butter or olive oil. And then with parmesan cheese or herb spices or feta.

NUTRITION (per serving): Calories: 157.3 kcal | Fats: 1.7g | Carbs: 8g | Protein: 6.7g.

25. FRENCH ONION SOUP

| 15 min | 45 min | Soft & Pureed food | 4 Servings |

INGREDIENTS

- 1 tbsp. olive oil
- 2 medium red or yellow onions, peeled and thinly sliced
- 1 leek, cleaned and thinly sliced
- 3½ cups beef stock
- 2 cloves garlic, minced
- ¼ tsp. thyme
- 1 tsp. Worcestershire sauce
- Salt and pepper, to taste
- 1 tbsp. Shredded cheese.

DIRECTIONS

1. In a medium pot, sauté onions and leeks until tender with olive oil over low-medium heat. Make sure not to burn the onion and leek. Stir in the garlic.

2. Add the beef stock and bring to boil.

3. Reduce heat. Cover and simmer for 30 minutes.

4. Turn off the heat and blend the soup.

5. Sprinkle shredded cheese for garnish.

6. Add salt and pepper to taste.

NUTRITION (per serving): Calories: 214 kcal | Fats: 21g | Carbs: 27g | Protein: 12g.

26. FRESH AVOCADO SOUP

| 5 min | 10 min | Soft & Pureed food | 2 Servings |

INGREDIENTS

- 1 ripe avocado
- 2 romaine lettuce leaves
- 1 cup coconut milk, chilled
- 1 tbsp. lime juice
- 20 fresh mint leaves.

DIRECTIONS

1. Mix all your ingredients thoroughly in a blender.

2. Chill in the fridge for 5-10 minutes.

NUTRITION (per serving): Calories: 280 kcal | Fats: 26g | Carbs: 2.6g | Protein: 4g

27. PUMPKIN SOUP

15 min

40 min

Soft & Pureed food

6 Servings

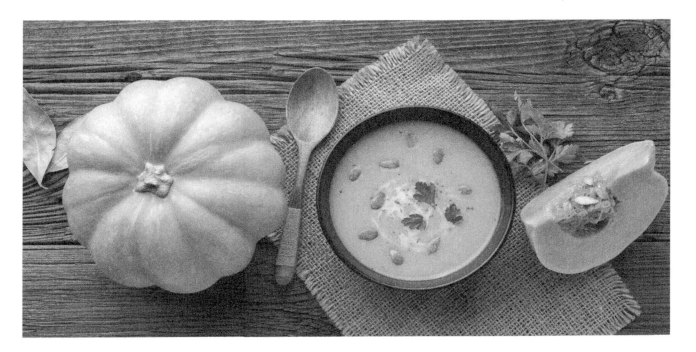

INGREDIENTS

- 1 tbsp. olive oil
- 1 medium onion, chopped
- 4 cloves garlic, minced
- 1 tbsp. ground cumin
- 1 tsp. chili powder
- ½ tsp. ground black pepper
- 2 cups vegetable broth
- 1 can (16 oz) of pumpkin purée (or roasted pumpkin).

DIRECTIONS

1. In a large pot, sauté onion, garlic, cumin, chili and pepper with olive oil until soft.

2. Add pumpkin puree and broth into the pot. Bring to boil. Stir occasionally.

3. Lower the heat with lid semi uncovered. Let the pumpkin soup simmer over low heat for 25 minutes.

4. Remove from heat. Use a blender to smoothen consistency.

5. Serve hot and enjoy!

NUTRITION (per serving): Calories: 230 kcal | Fats: 7g | Carbs: 35g | Protein: 9.8g.

28. CAULIFLOWER CHOWDER

| 15 min | 1 h | Soft & Pureed food | 6 Servings |

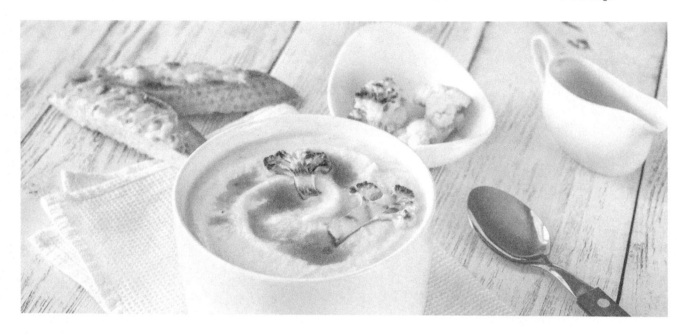

INGREDIENTS

- 1 tbsp. olive oil
- 3 cloves garlic, chopped
- 1 medium onion, chopped
- 3 medium carrots, chopped
- 3 cups cauliflower, chopped
- 3½ cups reduced sodium chicken broth
- 1 cup fat-free milk
- ¼ tsp. ground nutmeg
- ½ tsp. basil, dried
- 1 bay leaf
- Salt and pepper, to taste.

DIRECTIONS

1. In a large saucepan, sauté garlic and onion with olive oil until soft over low heat.

2. Add the remaining ingredients except the salt and pepper.

3. Bring to boil and let it simmer over low heat for additional 15 minutes. Season the soup with salt and pepper.

4. Remove from heat.

5. Blend the soup/chowder until smooth.

6. Bring it back to boil until the chowder is thickened. Stir occasionally.

7. Remove from heat. Serve hot.

NUTRITION (per serving): Calories: 195 kcal | Fats: 7g | Carbs: 31g | Protein: 9.2g.

29. CHEESY BROCCOLI SOUP

 10 min

 20 min

 Soft & Pureed food

 8 Servings

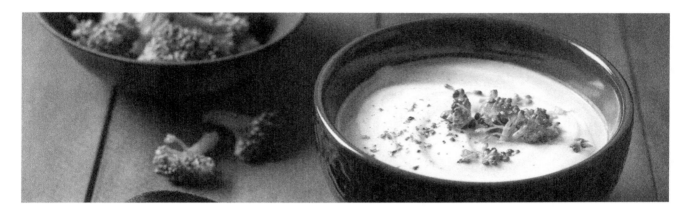

INGREDIENTS

- 1 tbsp. virgin olive oil
- 1 medium onion, chopped
- 1 tbsp. garlic, minced
- 2 cups carrots, grated
- ¼ tsp. ground nutmeg
- ¼ cup whole-wheat pastry flour
- 2 cups low-sodium vegetable broth
- 2 cups nonfat or 1% milk
- ½ cup fat-free half-and-half
- 3 cups broccoli florets
- 2 cups Cheddar cheese, shredded extra-sharp.

DIRECTIONS

1. In a stock pot, heat the olive oil over medium heat. Add the onion and garlic. Stir until fragrant, about 1 minute.

2. Add the carrots and continue to stir until tender, about 2 to 3 minutes. Add the nutmeg and the flour. Continue to cook, stirring constantly, until browned, 2 to 3 minutes.

3. Add the broth and then the milk and whisk constantly until it starts to thicken. Add the half-and-half and mix to combine well.

4. Stir in the broccoli florets. Bring to a boil and then reduce the heat to a simmer. Cook for 10 minutes or until the broccoli is tender.

5. Use an immersion blender to puree it to a smooth consistency, if desired, or leave it as is for a chunky soup.

6. Stir in the Cheddar cheese until melted. Reserve some cheese as a topping for serving time. Refrigerate any leftovers and eat within 1 week.

NUTRITION (per serving): Calories: 193 kcal | Fats: 9g | Carbs: 17g | Protein: 12g.

30. RED LENTIL SOUP WITH KALE

 10 min 45 min Soft & Pureed food 6 Servings

This Lentil Kale Soup is nutritious, delicious, vegan and protein-packed.

It's made with simple vegetables like onions, celery and carrots, loaded with plant-protein rich lentils and then finished off with some kale.

INGREDIENTS

- 1 tbsp. extra-virgin olive oil
- 1 cup onion, chopped
- ½ cup carrots, cut into ½-inch chunks
- ½ cup celery, cut into ¼-inch chunks
- 1 tsp. minced garlic
- 1 cup red lentils
- 1 tsp. thyme, dried
- 1 tsp. cumin, ground
- 2 cups low-sodium vegetable broth
- 2 cups water
- 2 large stalks kale, stemmed, with leaves chopped (about 2 cups)
- 1 bay leaf
- 2 tbsp. freshly squeezed lemon juice
- Low-fat plain Greek yogurt (optional).

DIRECTIONS

1. In a large stock pot over medium heat, heat the olive oil. Add the onion, carrots, celery, and garlic, and sauté until tender, 5 to 7 minutes.

2. Add the lentils, thyme, and cumin. Mix well and stir for 1 to 2 minutes until all the ingredients are coated well with the seasonings.

3. Add the broth and water to the pot. Bring to a simmer, add the kale, and stir well.

4. Add the bay leaf, then cover the pot and simmer for 30 to 35 minutes.

5. Remove the pot from the heat.

6. Remove and discard the bay leaf.

7. Stir in the lemon juice.

8. Use an immersion blender to puree the soup to your desired consistency. Alternatively, let the soup cool for 10 minutes before pureeing it in batches in a blender.

9. Garnish each bowl of soup with a dollop of the Greek yogurt (if using) and serve.

NUTRITION (per serving): Calories: 170 kcal | Fats: 3g | Carbs: 24g | Protein: 13g.

31. TURKEY CHILI

 5 min   25 min   Soft & Pureed food   6 Servings

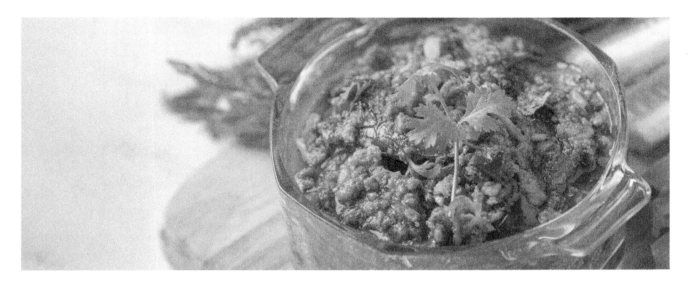

INGREDIENTS

- 1 lb. lean turkey meat, grounded
- 1½ tbsp. chilli powder
- 1 cup chicken broth
- 2 tbsp. olive oil
- 1 medium-sized onion, finely chopped
- 1½ tsp. cumin
- 1 can (or 28 oz.) pressed tomatoes
- 1 can kidney beans, rinsed and drained
- Ground pepper, to taste
- Salt, to taste.

DIRECTIONS

1. Place olive oil in a cooking pot and heat over medium temperature.

2. Sauté the onions and cook until softened.

3. Then add the turkey along with the spices.

4. Sauté until the turkey becomes brown.

5. Next, add the chicken broth and pressed tomatoes.

6. Close the lid of the cooking pot and cook for about 10 minutes.

7. Once the mixture obtains a pureed consistency, add the kidney beans and stir until it is softened.

8. Season it with ground pepper and a tiny pinch of salt.

NUTRITION (per serving): Calories: 335 kcal | Fats: 6.6g | Carbs: 41.3g | Protein: 21g.

32. WALNUT SQUASH PUREE

| 10 min | 1 h | Soft & Pureed food | 2 Servings |

INGREDIENTS

- 1 lb. squash, seeded and cut into large chunks
- 2 tbsp. olive oil

For spread:

- 3 tbsp. toasted walnuts, finely chopped
- ¼ medium onion, finely chopped
- ⅛ tsp. nutmeg, freshly grated
- 1 tsp. mint, freshly chopped
- ½ cup low-fat Parmesan cheese, grated
- Salt and pepper, to taste.

DIRECTIONS

SQUASH

1. Preheat the oven to 425°F.

2. Line a baking sheet with parchment or foil.

3. Place the squash on the baking sheet.

4. Rub the squash with 1 tablespoon of olive oil.

5. Bake for 45 minutes or until tender and fully cooked.

6. Remove from the oven and let the squash rest for 10 minutes.

7. Peel and discard the skin from squash.

8. Mash the squash with masher or fork. Set aside.

SPREAD

9. In a large skillet, sauté the onion in olive oil over medium-low heat.

10. Add salt, pepper, and cook the onion until tender, then remove from heat.

11. In a blender combine squash, onion, cheese, and all the remaining ingredients together.

12. Blend until smooth.

13. Add salt and pepper to taste.

NUTRITION (per serving): Calories: 226 kcal | Fats: 5.3g | Carbs: 32g | Protein: 8.4g.

33. CHEDDAR CHEESE PUFF

5 min

1 h

Soft & Pureed food

6 Servings

A flavorful, easy and soft cheesy protein meal that works for breakfast, lunch, supper, or as a tapas style appetizer! Melty cheddar provides the winning flavor for a make ahead bariatric-friendly meal your entire family will love.

INGREDIENTS

- 8 large eggs
- ⅓ cup flour
- 1 tsp. baking powder
- ½ tsp. salt
- Black pepper, to taste
- 1 cup, small curd low fat cottage cheese
- 1 cup Cheddar cheese, shredded
- 2 tbsp. butter, melted.

DIRECTIONS

1. Preheat the oven to 325°F.

2. Beat eggs until light and lemon colored - using an electric hand mixer if desired.

3. Add flour, baking powder, salt, a few grinds of black pepper and blend until smooth.

4. Fold in the cottage cheese, Cheddar cheese and butter.

5. Spray 8x8-inch glass baking dish with nonstick vegetable spray. Pour mixture into the baking dish.

6. Bake for 45 to 50 minutes, until edges are slightly puffed, and the very center of the puff still jiggles a bit when you move the baking dish.

7. DO NOT OVERBAKE - for a moist cheesy texture, remove from oven when slightly underbaked as the heat will continue to cook it out of the oven.

8. Allow to cool for 10 minutes.

9. Cut into squares and serve.

NUTRITION (per serving): Calories: 243 kcal | Fats: 19g | Carbs: 9.5g | Protein: 21g.

34. SIMPLE CREAMY GUACAMOLE

15 min

0 min

Soft & Pureed food

2 Servings

INGREDIENTS

- 1 ripe avocado, seeded and peeled
- 1 garlic clove, minced
- 1 tsp. lime or lemon juice
- ¼ tomato, finely chopped
- 1 tbsp. onion, chopped
- 1 tbsp. fresh cilantro leaves
- Salt, to taste.

DIRECTIONS

1. Put all the ingredients together in a blender.
2. Then blend them until smooth.
3. Serve immediately or refrigerate for an hour for best flavor.

NUTRITION (per serving): Calories: 109 kcal | Fats: 10g | Carbs: 6g | Protein: 1g.

35. HOMEMADE HUMMUS

10 min

0 min

Soft & Pureed food

6 Servings

INGREDIENTS

- 1 can (15 oz.) chickpeas
- ½ cup hot water
- 2 garlic cloves
- 2 tbsp. sesame seeds
- ¼ tsp. parsley
- ¼ tsp. ground red paprika
- 1 tbsp. lemon juice
- 1 tbsp. olive oil
- Salt and pepper, to taste.

DIRECTIONS

1. In a blender add sesame seeds, olive oil and lemon juice. Blend until smooth.
2. Then add all the other ingredients and blend until smooth.
3. Season hummus with salt and pepper to taste.

NUTRITION (per serving): Calories: 166 kcal | Fats: 9.6g | Carbs: 14.3g | Protein: 7.9g.

36. EGG CUSTARD WITH BERRIES

5 min

50 min

Soft & Pureed food

4 Servings

Egg Custard is a wonderful delicious soft dish of cool vanilla creaminess and berry flavor. Easy smooth and creamy. It is the most perfect bariatric food for all post ops.

INGREDIENTS

- 2 large-sized eggs
- 1 cup blueberries
- 1 cup raspberries
- ¼ tsp. nutmeg
- 1 tsp. vanilla extract
- 4 tsp. sugar substitute
- 1 cup water
- 2 cups evaporated milk, nonfat
- ¼ tsp. salt.

DIRECTIONS

1. Heat the oven until it reached 350°F.

2. Pour in water in a baking pan with a measurement of 9x13 inches.

3. Also, prepare an 8x8 baking dish and spray it with nonstick cooking spray.

4. Prepare a small bowl, then place sugar substitute, a pinch of salt, vanilla extract, and eggs.

5. Beat them thoroughly until all ingredients are diluted.

6. Next is to pour the nonfat evaporated milk. Stir the mixture until blended well.

7. Mix and shake raspberries and blueberries. And then place them at the bottom of the 8x8 baking pan—spread them evenly throughout.

8. Then put the egg mixture on top.

9. Next, transfer the ingredients of the 8x8 pan into the water-filled 9x13 pan.

10. Bake and wait for another 35 minutes, or until no crumbs are sticking to the knife when you put it in.

11. Remove the baking pan from the oven.

12. Lastly, sprinkle nutmeg on top of the custard.

NUTRITION (per serving): Calories: 140 kcal | Fats: 5g | Carbs: 45g | Protein: 14.2g.

37. VANILLA EGG CUSTARD

 10 min

 50 min

 Soft & Pureed food

 4 Servings

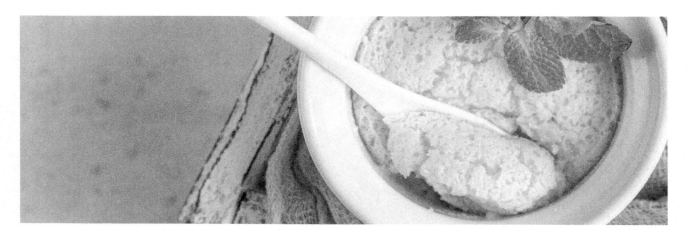

INGREDIENTS

- 1 cup low-fat milk
- 1 (12 oz.) can evaporated low-fat milk
- 4 large eggs
- ⅔ cup Splenda
- 2 tsp. vanilla extract
- Freshly grated nutmeg.

DIRECTIONS

1. Preheat oven to 325°F.

2. Place 6 custard cups or ramekins in a large roasting pan and set aside.

3. Combine the milk, evaporated milk, eggs, vanilla and Splenda in the blender and pulse 3-4 times until smooth.

4. Pour into the custard cups and grate a bit of nutmeg over each one.

5. Pour enough hot water in the roasting pan to come about halfway up the sides of the custards and bake 25 to 35 minutes, until just set in the center and are still a little jiggly.

6. Before removing from oven, make sure your custards have set - oven temps and size of custard cups vary.

7. Carefully remove the custards from the water bath, and transfer to towel. Let cool. Serve chilled.

NUTRITION (per serving): Calories: 140 kcal | Fats: 5g | Carbs: 45g | Protein: 14.2g.

38. COTTAGE CHEESE FLUFF RECIPE

10 min

0 min

Soft & Pureed food

4 Servings

INGREDIENTS

- 24 oz. fat-free cottage cheese
- 4 oz. sugar-free whipped crème
- 1 (0.3 oz.) packages sugar-free gelatin, flavor of choice
- Fruits (optional).

DIRECTIONS

1. Mix all ingredients in a medium bowl.
2. Optional — add your favorite fruit pureed in a blender.

NUTRITION (per serving): Calories: 220 kcal | Fats: 3g | Carbs: 24g | Protein: 22g.

39. CHEESECAKE PUDDING RECIPE

5 min

0 min

Soft & Pureed food

1 Servings

INGREDIENTS

- 1 cup plain fat-free Greek yogurt
- 1 package sugar-free cheesecake pudding mix.

DIRECTIONS

1. Combine all the ingredients in a blender.
2. Puree until smooth.

NUTRITION (per serving): Calories: 67 kcal | Fats: 0g | Carbs: 1g | Protein: 7g.

40. PUMPKIN YOGURT WITH EXTRA KICK

10 min

0 min

Soft & Pureed food

2 Servings

INGREDIENTS

- ½ cup pumpkin, canned
- ¼ tsp. cinnamon
- ⅛ tsp. all-spice
- ⅛ tsp. nutmeg
- ⅛ tsp. ground ginger
- 1 cup vanilla yogurt (light)
- 1 tsp. vanilla extract
- Stevia, to taste
- ½ tsp. liquid butter extract.

DIRECTIONS

1. Combine all ingredients and mix thoroughly.
2. Place in a refrigerator and chill for a few minutes before serving.

NUTRITION (per serving): Calories: 30 kcal | Fats: 0.1g | Carbs: 8g | Protein: 1,2g.

41. ORANGE APPLE POPSICLES

5 min

0 min

Soft & Pureed food

2 Servings

INGREDIENTS

- 3 fresh oranges, peeled and pith removed
- 2 large apples, peeled, corked and halved.

DIRECTIONS

1. Blend all the ingredients together until smooth.
2. Pour the juice into the popsicle mold or mini paper cups.
3. Freeze overnight.

NUTRITION (per serving): Calories: 135 kcal | Fats: 0g | Carbs: 22g | Protein: 1g.

42. BERRIES YOGURT POPSICLE

10 min	0 min	Soft & Pureed food	3 Servings

INGREDIENTS

- 1 cup blueberries, washed and cleaned
- 1 cup blackberries, washed and cleaned
- 1 packet Stevia sugar
- 1 cup low-fat vanilla yogurt.

DIRECTIONS

1. Blend blueberries and blackberries until smooth. Then strain the puree mixture for a smoother consistency.

2. Add stevia into the berries puree. Mix well.

3. Prepare the popsicle molds. Pour the berries puree, equally, into each mold, and topped with yogurt. Freeze overnight.

NUTRITION (per serving): Calories: 65 kcal | Fats: 5g | Carbs: 12g | Protein: 3g.

43. PROTEIN POPSICLES

5 min	0 min	Soft & Pureed food	4 Servings

INGREDIENTS

- 2 cups fresh or frozen strawberries, washed and stem removed
- 1 medium ripe banana, peeled and sliced
- 1 cup of pre-made clear protein drinks of your choice.

DIRECTIONS

1. Blend all the ingredients together until smooth.

2. Divide the mixture equally in popsicles mold.

3. Freeze overnight.

NUTRITION (per serving): Calories: 57 kcal | Fats: 2g | Carbs: 25g | Protein: 26g.

Chapter 6

INTRODUCING REAL FOODS

HOW MUCH CAN I EAT AFTER SURGERY?

Now that we have had a chance to talk about some of the basics of this diet plan and how it works, it is time for us to dive into the amount of food or how much we can put into a serving when the surgery is done. We want to be able to lose weight, so obviously the serving sizes need to be smaller, but we want to make sure that we are eating enough to meet our nutrition needs while not eating so much that we are going to end up straining the stomach and causing injury after this kind of surgery.

When the surgery is done, you want to make sure that you are careful with the amount that you are eating. During the liquid phase and the time before the diet where you are not supposed to eat at all, hopefully, you will start to recognize the difference between having cravings and wanting to eat versus being hungry and actually needing to eat. The more that you are able to learn how to do that, the easier the weight loss will be, and the easier it is for the recovery time after the sleeve as well.

With this in mind, we need to take it slowly and learn how to listen to our bodies. Going back to some of the old ways of doing things and our old eating habits will be hard to do here because the sleeve is going to slow that down. But if you are not careful, over time, the stomach will stretch out, and you will start to take on more food than you should, and the weight will come back. That is why we need to learn how to listen to our bodies and what they tell us as early as possible.

During the first few weeks, you do not have to worry as much about the portions as you will with the other parts. This is the time where you are mostly going to have water and not much else. Your goal is to give the stomach some time to heal, and lots of water is going to be your best friend. Towards the second week, you are able to add in some light things, think the foods you would eat when suffering from a big cold, and the amounts that you would eat during that time as well. But during that first week, you will focus on keeping just with the liquids and maybe some broth if you are feeling a bit hungry.

During the second week, you will not increase your food amounts that much either. You will be allowed to add in a few things like yogurt, pudding, and maybe even a few easy to consume soups as long as they have a ton of nutrition in them. The servings need to stay pretty small. Think like one small pudding cup for breakfast, one small yogurt for lunch, and a kid's bowl of soup for supper, followed with water for the rest of the day. And that is only if you feel up to it. If even that much food is still not sitting well with you, then taper it back and keep things small.

After those first few weeks, your stomach should be feeling better, and if you followed the diet in the right manner you will then be able to increase your portions a bit and eat a little bit more. But you still need to be careful and worry about what is going to feel the best for you here.

The foods that you eat during this time need to be soft and easy to digest because you are only a bit past that mark of having the surgery, and you want to make sure that your stomach is getting the healing that it needs. Lots of soft fruits and vegetables are encouraged here, and just having a little bit is a good place to start. If you are worried about servings, a good idea is to replace all of your dishes, at least for now, with some of the plates that are made for toddlers. The ones that separate out into a few sections can be even better.

This way you can fill up that little plate and know when you are done and should not eat anymore. These will keep some of the meals that you consume down to a minimum and will make it easier for some self-control. In these weeks, your body will be adjusting to some of the changes that you have made, and you want to make sure that you aren't overloading it too much. Starting with some smaller portions is a great way to make sure that we are going to keep our bodies healthy, get the nutrients that we need, and allow for the rest of the healing that is needed.

As you are eating during this stage, and any of the other stages that you work with, you want to make sure that you are eating nice and slow. If you scarf down the meal, you risk eating too much along the way, and you are going to definitely feel it when the time is all done. This is not a healthy way to eat whether you are on this kind of diet plan or not, so avoid it as much as possible and build up some slower eating habits.

It is recommended, especially in the beginning, that you chew your food 25 times before swallowing. If you are still in the first few weeks of eating solid foods, although this may be a bit hard to do with some blended and pureed foods, so don't worry about that as much. But taking your time is going to be so important when you work on this kind of plan and being careful with not scarfing down the food will allow you time to know when you are hungry and can reduce complications from eating too much and tearing the stomach.

If it is too hard to eat the food and take in that many bites at a time, then set a timer for how long you will take to eat the meal. Maybe give yourself 20 minutes to get the plate done. If you feel full before that time, then stop eating, no matter how much is already on the plate still, but make sure that the plate is not empty before the timer goes off.

During this time, you should only eat three meals a day, and the snacking should definitely be limited as much as possible. This will ensure that you are not going to end up with issues of grazing and eating too much as the day goes on and that you can monitor your calories as you go. As you get more familiar with this eating plan, and you are sure that you can handle it all, you can then go through and add in some more foods and meals as well, and maybe have a snack on occasion. But in the beginning, stick with the three meals a day and do not go back for seconds, or you could cause issues.

Eating is going to be a bit trickier to manage when you are on this kind of diet plan compared to some of the others that you may have done in the past. You are not only learning how to cut down the calories and listen to your body for the actual hunger cues that will tell you when to eat. You also need to worry about the healing process and not eat too much as you go through this. All of that combined is going to be a bit harder to stick with when you first get started, but it can be a great way to ensure that you can lose weight and keep that weight off for the long term as well.

SOLID FOODS

(From 2 to 3 months and onwards) After 2 or 3 months, you can go back to eating solid foods. But after such, you can feel changes in your appetite and find that you become full quicker before the surgery.

Although you may eat more solid foods at this point, it doesn't mean that you're allowed to somewhat careless in what you eat. The following are some examples of foods that are still off-limits during this phase:

- Tough meat – be sure to tenderize or marinade them before consuming.

- Bread – we prefer for you to toast and slice them first.

- High-fat and high-calorie milk products – we advise low-lactose milk and soya milk instead.

Important notes:

- Strictly comply with the diet guidelines provided by your dietician or surgeon.

- Stop eating as soon as you feel full.

- Take time to consume your meals.

- Chew your foods thoroughly.

- Opt for chewable dietary supplements. However, in events, you can't find any crush tablet supplements or pour in water if in capsule form.

- Never skip meals. Eat three times a day.

You may still experience nausea and vomiting from time to time. But as soon as you start experiencing them, stop eating.

Chapter 7

BREAKFAST RECIPES

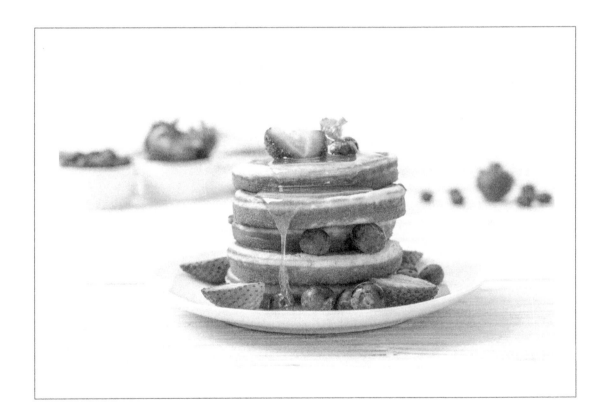

44. CHERRY-VANILLA BAKED OATMEAL

| 10 min | 45 min | Breakfast | 6 Servings |

INGREDIENTS

- 3 medium eggs
- 1 cup old-fashioned oats
- 1 tbsp. flaxseed powder
- 1 tsp. vanilla extract
- ½ tsp. cinnamon powder
- 1 cup low-fat milk
- 1 tsp. liquid stevia
- ¾ tsp. baking powder
- 1 medium apple, diced cored and skinless
- ½ cup low-fat plain greek yogurt
- 1 cup fresh cherries with the pits removed
- Nonstick cooking spray.

DIRECTIONS

1. Prepare your oven. Preheat to 375°F.
2. Grease an 8x8 inch baking dish with nonstick cooking spray.
1. Get a medium bowl. Pour in cinnamon powder, flaxseed, oats, and baking powder into it. Mix thoroughly and set aside.
2. In a much larger bowl, crack the eggs and whisk.

   Then add yogurt, stevia, milk, and vanilla. Whisk again until thoroughly mixed.
3. Stir the dry ingredients into the wet ingredients.
4. Now pour in diced apples and cherries, then gently fold them into the mixture.
5. Pour mixture into the prepared baking dish and slide it into the oven to bake.
6. Leave it for about 45 minutes or until you notice the edges pulling away from the walls of the pan and the oatmeal bouncing back when poked.
7. Place any leftovers into airtight glass bowls and place them in the fridge. They will keep for a week. Microwave before serving

Notes: Play around with the extras in the oatmeal. In fact, make the recipes seasonal even. Change it up every now and then. Use pumpkin puree in place of the yogurt. Use unsweetened dried cranberries instead of the usual cherries if you'd like a nice holiday twist. Place the apples and cherries on the shelf and replace them with 100% natural fresh berries. If you would like a super creamy consistency, you can add a quarter cup of low-fat milk when serving.

NUTRITION (per serving): Calories: 149 kcal | Fats: 4g | Carbs: 21g | Protein: 8g.

45. HEARTY SLOW COOKER CINNAMON OATMEAL

5 min

8 h

Breakfast

10 Servings

INGREDIENTS

- 2 cups steel-cut oats
- 1 tsp. nutmeg powder
- 8 cups water
- 2 tsp. cinnamon powder
- Protein add-ins for 8 weeks post-op (use one at a time)
- 2 tbsp. vanilla or unflavored protein powder
- 2 tbsp. peanut butter powder
- ½ cup low-fat milk
- 2 tbsp. nonfat milk powder or powdered egg white
- ¼ cup pumpkin puree
- ½ cup frozen or fresh berries
- ⅛ cup walnuts, almonds, or pecans, chopped
- ½ medium pear, banana or apple, peeled

DIRECTIONS

1. Pour oats, water, nutmeg, and cinnamon powder into a slow cooker.

2. Put a lid on it and place it over l9w heat to simmer for about 8 hours or 7, give or take.

3. You have quite a number of protein add-ins to pick from. Choose one and stir it into the mixture right before serving. Feel free to change it up anytime you like.

Notes: A quick tip, oatmeal is packed with soluble fiber needed for topnotch heart health. All foods that contain soluble fiber have been tested and trusted to reduce the bad cholesterol in your blood, leading to a healthy heart and healthier you. If you're in need of a quick, healthy, and filling breakfast, go for oatmeal.

NUTRITION (per serving): Calories: 136 kcal | Fats: 2g | Carbs: 23g | Protein: 6g.

46. HIGH-PROTEIN PANCAKES

 5 min

 5 min

 Breakfast

 4 Servings

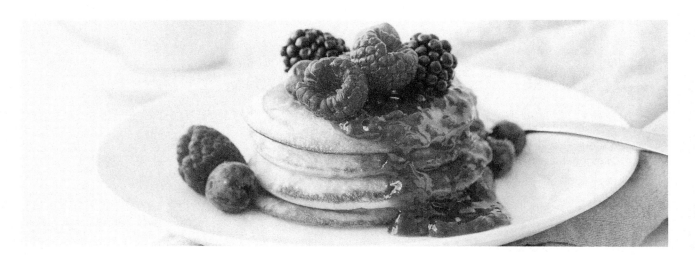

INGREDIENTS

- 1½ tbsp. melted coconut oil
- 3 medium eggs
- ⅓ cup whole wheat pastry flour
- 1 cup low-fat cottage cheese
- Nonstick cooking spray.

DIRECTIONS

1. Gently beat the eggs in a large bowl.

2. Stir in flour, coconut oil, and cottage cheese until thoroughly mixed.

3. Place a large pan over medium-low heat and grease the pan with a single coat of cooking spray.

4. You will need a measuring cup for this part. Drizzle about ⅓ cup of pancake batter into a greased pan and leave it to cook for about 3 minutes or until you notice air bubbles on top of the pancake.

5. Flip the pancakes to cook the other side until it looks golden brown. This should take about 2 minutes. Take it out of the pan and repeat the process until the batter is finished.

6. Serve warm.

NUTRITION (per serving): Calories: 182 kcal | Fats: 10g | Carbs: 10g | Protein: 12g.

47. COTTAGE CHEESE PANCAKES

15 min

30 min

Breakfast

6 Servings

INGREDIENTS

- ¾ cup flour
- ½ tsp. baking soda
- ¼ tsp. salt
- 1 tbsp. stevia (optional)
- 2 eggs
- ¾ cup low-fat cottage cheese
- ½ cup nonfat milk
- Nonstick cooking spray.

DIRECTIONS

1. In a large bowl, whisk all ingredients together.
2. Lightly coat a skillet or griddle with cooking spray.
3. Place about 2 tablespoons of the batter into the skillet.
4. Cook the pancakes over medium heat for 2-3 minutes on each side or until golden brown and cooked in the center.
5. Serve warm.

NUTRITION (per serving): Calories: 197 kcal | Fats: 12g | Carbs: 9.8g | Protein: 14g.

48. FLOURLESS PANCAKES

10 min

20 min

Breakfast

6 Servings

INGREDIENTS

- 2 large eggs
- 2 ripe bananas, mashed
- ½ tsp. cinnamon (optional)
- 1 tsp. vanilla extract
- ⅛ tsp. baking powder
- Pinch of salt
- 1 tbsp. olive oil
- Nonstick cooking spray.

DIRECTIONS

1. Combine all ingredients in a bowl.
2. Lightly coat the non-stick skillet with cooking spray.
3. Pour 2 tablespoons of batter into the skillet. Cook over medium-low heat until small bubbles are formed.
4. Flip the pancake. It may take about 2 minutes to cook on each side.

NUTRITION (per serving): Calories: 197 kcal | Fats: 15g | Carbs: 6.1g | Protein: 11.5g.

49. FRENCH CHEESE CREPES

25 min

25 min

Breakfast

10 Servings

INGREDIENTS

For crepes skin

- 2 eggs
- ¾ cup of nonfat milk
- 1 tbsp. of olive oil
- ½ cup of flour.

For filling

- ¾ cup of low-fat small curd cottage cheese, drained
- 2 tsp. of splenda
- 1 tbsp. of lemon juice.

DIRECTIONS

TO MAKE CREPES SKIN:

1. Whisk together all ingredients in a medium bowl. Try to reduce lumps.

2. Use the crepes maker (follow the manufacturer instructions) or using a non-stick skillet over medium heat.

3. Pour batter about 2 tablespoons per crepe into the skillet.

4. Cook the batter for 1 -2 minutes for each side.

TO MAKE COTTAGE CHEESE FILLING:

5. Combine all of the ingredients listed for making filling. Mix well.

TO FILL AND ROLL THE CREPES:

6. Take a layer of the crepe skin. Place about 1- 2 tablespoons of filling in the center.

7. Fold the right and left edges toward the center.

8. Roll the crepe to seal the filling in. Set it aside.

9. Repeat until all the crepes are filled. You can store the filled crepes in the refrigerator.

TO COOK THE CREPES:

10. Over medium- high heat, coat the pan with one teaspoon of oil or butter.

11. Add crepe(s). Cook until brown and crispy for about 2 minutes per side. Serve warm.

NUTRITION (per serving): Calories: 197 kcal | Fats: 17g | Carbs: 12g | Protein: 16g.

50. RICOTTA BERRY PIE

 10 min   35 min   Breakfast   6 Servings

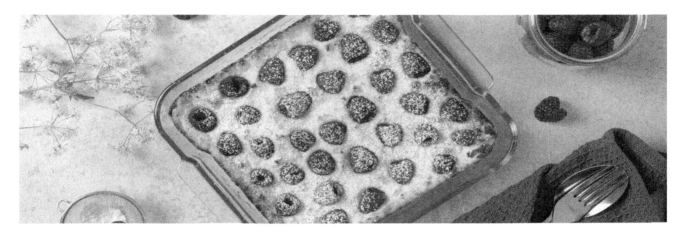

INGREDIENTS

- 3 eggs
- ½ cup Stevia
- 1 tsp. pure vanilla extract
- 1 (15 oz.) container part skim ricotta cheese
- ½ cup fresh blackberries, raspberries or blueberries.

DIRECTIONS

1. Preheat oven to 325°F.

2. Using the blender, pulse the eggs, Stevia, vanilla and ricotta until smooth.

3. Pour filling into pie plate that has been coated with vegetable non stick spray.

4. Drop the berries decoratively into the custard.

5. Bake for 30 to 35 minutes, until the filling is slightly puffed at the edges, barely golden and just set - meaning it should be slightly jiggly in the center when you gently move the pie plate from side to side - a little soft in the center is desired. DO NOT OVERBAKE.

6. Remove from the oven and let cool on a rack. Serve at room temperature or chilled.

NUTRITION (per serving): Calories: 204 kcal | Fats: 23g | Carbs: 17g | Protein: 8.2g.

51. NO SUGAR FRENCH YOGURT CAKE

 5 min

 1 h 5 min

 Breakfast

 10 Servings

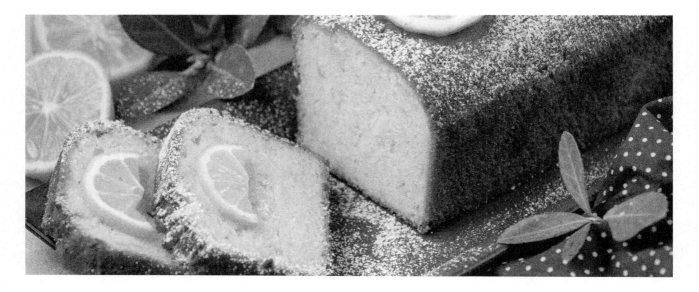

INGREDIENTS

- ¾ cup almond flour
- ¾ cup all purpose flour
- 2 tsp. baking powder
- ½ tsp. sea salt
- ½ cup Stevia sugar
- ½ cup plain yogurt
- 4 tbsp. butter, melted
- 2 large eggs
- 1 lemon zest, freshly grated
- ½ lemon juice
- 1 tsp. vanilla extract.

DIRECTIONS

1. Preheat oven to 350°F.
2. Coat a loaf pan with non-stick vegetable spray.
3. Whisk together to combine in small bowl the almond flour, flour, baking powder, salt - set aside.
4. In a large bowl, with your fingers, rub together the lemon zest and Stevia.
5. Whisk in the yogurt, butter, eggs, lemon juice and vanilla extract.
6. Blend in the flour mixture.
7. Transfer into loaf pan and smooth top.
8. Bake 40 to 45 minutes, until golden brown, top has risen, and thin skewer inserted near center comes out clean.
9. Let cool on wire rack for 15 minutes, invert onto rack and cool completely.

NUTRITION (per serving): Calories: 204 kcal | Fats: 23g | Carbs: 17g | Protein: 8.2g.

52. PROTEIN WAFFLE

5 min

10 min

Breakfast

2 Servings

INGREDIENTS

- 1 egg, lightly beaten
- 1 tbsp. almond milk
- 1 scoop protein powder
- ¼ tsp. baking powder, gluten-free
- 1 tbsp. butter, melted
- ¼ tsp. salt.

DIRECTIONS

1. Incorporate all ingredients in a bowl.

2. Spray waffle maker with cooking spray.

3. Pour half of the mix in waffle maker and cook until golden brown. Repeat.

NUTRITION (per serving): Calories: 160 kcal | Fats: 10.7g | Carbs: 2.7g | Protein: 18.9g.

53. BANANA MUFFIN IN A MUG

5 min

30 sec

Breakfast

1 Servings

INGREDIENTS

- 1 scoop protein powder
- 1 tbsp. plain non-fat yogurt or no sugar added applesauce (this will add moisture)
- ½ tsp. baking powder.

DIRECTIONS

1. In a Vented Microwave Cup, mix protein, yogurt or applesauce, baking powder and milk into smooth paste.

2. Close the lid on the mug and open the vent on the top.

3. Cook in microwave for 20 - 30 seconds. DO NOT OVERCOOK.

4. Cake will continue to cook once removed from microwave. Should be slightly molten and jiggle a bit.

Notes: You may top this with 3-4 very thin slices of a small banana.

NUTRITION (per serving): Calories: 197 kcal | Fats: 9.2g | Carbs: 6.9g | Protein: 21.8g.

54. SOUTHWESTERN SCRAMBLED EGGS BURRITOS

 10 min

 10 min

 Breakfast

 8 Servings

INGREDIENTS

- 1 tsp. extra-virgin olive oil
- 1 medium red bell pepper, chopped
- 1 medium green bell pepper, chopped
- ¼ cup low-fat milk
- 8 medium whole wheat tortillas
- 12 small eggs
- 1 can black beans, drained and rinsed
- 1 cup salsa
- ½ medium onion, diced.

DIRECTIONS

1. Mix the eggs and milk in a large bowl.

2. Place a large pan over medium heat and drizzle olive oil onto it.

3. Pour in bell peppers, and onions, then stir-fry for about 3 minutes or until it softens.

4. Stir in the beans.

5. Pour in the milk mixture and lower the heat to a simmer and gently stir with a silicone spatula for roughly 4 minutes or until the eggs look cooked through and fluffy.

6. Place the tortillas on a clean flat surface and scoop the scrambled egg mixture onto each of them.

7. Fold the tortilla. Bottom end first, then the sides, then roll.

8. Serve warm with a side of salsa.

Notes: Place any leftovers in the fridge to preserve. This will keep for a week. To serve, microwave for 1 minute and 30 seconds.

If you want to store them for longer than a week, you will have to put them on ice.

NUTRITION (per serving): Calories: 250 kcal | Fats: 10g | Carbs: 28g | Protein: 19g.

55. HARD-BOILED EGGS AND AVOCADO

20 min

10 min

Breakfast

2 Servings

INGREDIENTS

- 1 Avocado
- 4 slices of sprouted bread
- 4 eggs
- 1 tsp. hot sauce
- Salt and pepper, to taste.

DIRECTIONS

1. Cook the eggs in a boiling water for 10 minutes, then let cool.
2. Meanwhile toast the bread and mash the avocado with a fork in a bowl and mix in the hot sauce.
3. Peel the eggs and slice into fourths going lengthwise.
4. Spread this mash over the four slices of toast and then top with the egg slices. Add salt and pepper before serving.

NUTRITION (per serving): Calories: 191 kcal | Fats: 15g | Carbs: 10g | Protein: 10g.

56. WISCONSIN SCRAMBLER

20 min

10 min

Breakfast

6 Servings

INGREDIENTS

- 3 oz. cheddar cheese, wisconsin
- ½ tsp. garlic powder
- ½ tsp. onion powder
- ¼ cup low-fat milk
- 6 beaten eggs
- 8 oz. turkey sausage, lean
- Cooking spray.

DIRECTIONS

1. In a skillet cook the turkey sausage and brown it with a wooden spoon, breaking into smaller pieces to cook it all through.
2. In a bowl on the side, whisk together the milk and eggs. Mix in the garlic powder and onion.
3. Add the eggs to the skillet and reduce the heat a bit. Stir gently and all the time with a rubber spatula. Continue until the eggs are cooked all the way through.
4. Top with some cheese and then serve.

NUTRITION (per serving): Calories: 169 kcal | Fats: 2g | Carbs: 11g | Protein: 15g.

57. HANGRY EGGS

10 min

20 min

Breakfast

6 Servings

INGREDIENTS

- 2 eggs
- 4 slices deli ham
- ½ bag cauliflower florets
- Cooking spray.

DIRECTIONS

1. Place the cauliflower and 2 tablespoons of water into a bowl and cover in the microwave for 4 minutes to make tender.

2. In the last half a minute, add the ham to this and heat it through. If there is water left, drain it out when you are done.

3. Coat a skillet with some cooking spray and place it on medium heat. When the skillet is nice and hot, add the eggs and reduce the heat a bit. You will know it is done when the whites start to turn opaque and the yolks start to cook, but it is still soft in the middle.

4. Place the cauliflower on a plate and have the ham on top. Add the eggs over it all, and then serve.

NUTRITION (per serving): Calories: 109 kcal | Fats: 4g | Carbs: 6g | Protein: 11g.

58. OMELET IN A CUP

5 min

5 min

Breakfast

1 Servings

INGREDIENTS

- 1 large egg
- 1 tbsp. water
- Salt and paper, to taste
- Cooking spray.

DIRECTIONS

1. Lightly coat a microwave-safe cup with cooking spray.

2. In a cup, beat egg, water, salt and pepper with a fork. Mix well.

3. Cook in a microwave for 60 seconds or until egg is fully cooked.

NUTRITION (per serving): Calories: 109 kcal | Fats: 4g | Carbs: 6g | Protein: 11g.

59. GRUYÈRE & PARMESAN SOUFFLÉ

25 min

35 min

Breakfast

5 Servings

INGREDIENTS

- 4 large eggs, separate the yolks from the whites
- 2½ tbsp. unsalted butter
- 3 tbsp. flour
- ½ tsp. garlic powder
- ½ tsp. salt
- ½ tsp. cream of tartar
- ⅛ tsp. black pepper
- ¼ tsp. dry mustard powder
- Pinch of nutmeg
- 1 cup nonfat milk
- 1 cup low-fat Gruyère (or Cheddar, or Swiss cheese), shredded
- ½ cup Parmesan, shredded.

DIRECTIONS

1. Preheat the oven to 375°F.

2. Grease the ramekin with butter. Set aside.

3. Warm milk in a saucepan over medium-low heat right before boiling. Do not burn the milk.

4. Make the roux (butter and flour mixture): Melt butter in a saucepan over medium heat. Add flour and whisk until mixture begins to bubble, do not allow mixture to brown. Remove saucepan from heat.

5. Let the roux stand for few minutes to cool. Pour in warm milk, whisking until smooth. Return to heat.

6. Whisk the mixture of roux and milk constantly until thick, for about 2 to 3 minutes. Remove from heat.

7. Add black pepper, salt, and nutmeg. Add egg yolks one at a time, whisking to blend after each addition.

8. Scrape the mixture into large bowl and let it rest at room temperature.

9. Use a mixer to beat egg whites in another large bowl for 3 minutes. Then add cream of tartar, mix again until the egg whites form a stiff peak.

10. Fold ¼ of whites into lukewarm or room temperature mixture. Do not over mix. Add the cheese along with egg whites.

11. Transfer the soufflé mixture to prepared ramekin.

12. Place ramekin in the oven for 35 minutes or until soufflé is puffed and golden brown on top. Do not open the oven for the first 20 minutes or the batter will deflate.

NUTRITION (per serving): Calories: 312 kcal | Fats: 27.1g | Carbs: 15.4g | Protein: 22.8g.

60. BERRY CHIA PUDDING

 10 min   1 h   Breakfast   4 Servings

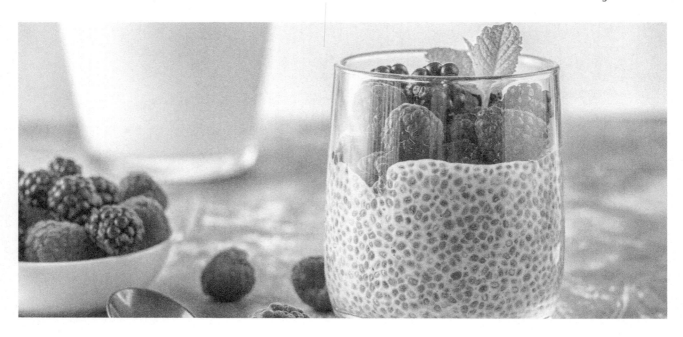

INGREDIENTS

- 3 cups coconut milk (canned full-fat)
- ½ cup berries
- 2 tbsp. vanilla protein powder
- 2 pinches sea salt
- 8 tbsp. chia seeds.

Toppings (optional)

- Blueberries
- Strawberries
- Banana

DIRECTIONS

1. In a high-speed blender, add the coconut milk, the berries and the protein powder. Also add two pinches of salt to balance the flavor. Blend until smooth!

2. In a large bowl, add chia seeds and then pour the berry coconut milk on top and stir well.

3. Put it in the refrigerator overnight (or at least 1 hour).

4. Right before serving, dish up and add your toppings of choice. You can use cut or smooth berries and fruits. Enjoy!

NUTRITION (per serving): Calories: 152 kcal | Fats: 22.5g | Carbs: 5.7g | Protein: 7.1g.

Chapter 8

ENTREES & SNACKS RECIPES

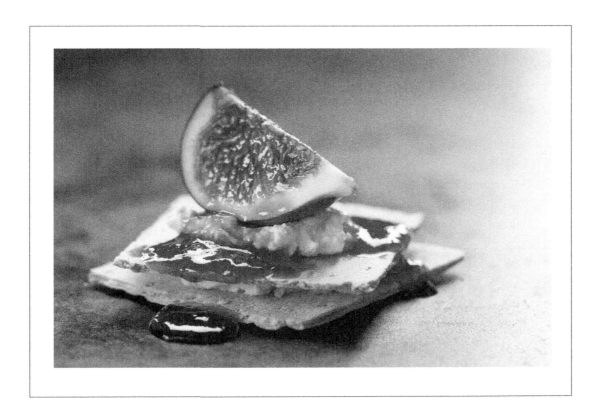

61. SOUTHWEST DEVILED EGGS

10 min

10 min

Entrees & Snacks

6 Servings

INGREDIENTS

- 6 large eggs, hard-boiled
- 2 tbsp. low-fat, plain Greek yogurt
- ¼ tsp. spicy mustard
- ⅛ tsp. salt
- ½ tsp. Taco seasoning.

DIRECTIONS

1. Peel the eggs and halve them lengthwise.
2. Remove the yolks, and transfer them to a small bowl, setting the whites aside.
3. Add the yogurt, spicy mustard, salt, and taco seasoning to the bowl with the yolks, and mash everything together.
4. Spoon or pipe egg yolk mixture into egg halves. Cover and chill at least 1 hour or until ready to serve. Garnish, if desired.

NUTRITION (per serving): Calories: 83 kcal | Fats: 5g | Carbs: 1g | Protein: 7g.

62. CHEESE JALAPENO MUFFINS

10 min

20 min

Entrees & Snacks

12 Servings

INGREDIENTS

- Cooking spray, for pan
- 9 eggs
- 6 bacon slices
- ¾ cup heavy cream
- 1½ jalapeno pepper, sliced
- 8.5 oz. cheddar cheese, shredded
- Pepper
- Salt.

DIRECTIONS

1. Preheat the oven to 350°F. Prep muffin tray with cooking spray and add cooked bacon slices to each muffin cup.
2. In a large bowl, whisk together eggs, cheese, cream, pepper, and salt.
3. Pour egg mixture into the prepared muffin tray.
4. Add sliced jalapeno into each muffin cup.
5. Bake for 15-20 minutes.

NUTRITION (per serving): Calories: 28 kcal | Fats: 2.4g | Carbs: 1g | Protein: 6.4g.

63. CAPRESE SALAD BITES

 10 min 15 min Entrees & Snacks 12 Servings

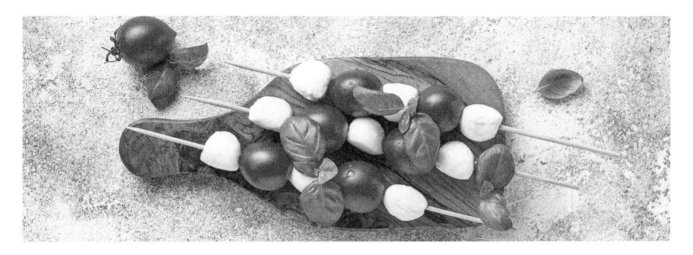

INGREDIENTS

- 24 cherry tomatoes
- 12 mozzarella balls
- 12 fresh basil leaves.

For the Balsamic Glaze

- ½ cup balsamic vinegar
- 2 tbsp. extra-virgin olive oil
- 1 garlic clove, minced
- 1 tsp. Italian seasoning.

DIRECTIONS

TO MAKE THE BITES

1. Using 12 toothpicks or short skewers, assemble each with 1 cherry tomato, 1 mozzarella ball, 1 basil leaf, and another tomato.

2. Place on a serving platter or in a large glass storage container that can be sealed.

TO MAKE THE GLAZE

3. In a small saucepan, bring the balsamic to a simmer. Simmer for 15 minutes, or until syrupy. Set aside to cool and thicken.

4. In a small bowl, whisk olive oil, garlic, Italian seasoning, and cooled vinegar.

5. Drizzle the olive oil and balsamic glaze over the skewers. Serve immediately or keep in the refrigerator for a tasty snack.

NUTRITION (per serving): Calories: 23 kcal | Fats: 2g | Carbs: 0.4g | Protein: 2g.

64. SHRIMP STUFFED AVOCADOS

15 min

2 min

Entrees & Snacks

4 Servings

Shrimp and avocado are a match made in heaven. Beautifully ripe avocado is a fat in this dish - it replaces the mayonnaise!

There is not a recipe for this one as it's that easy!

INGREDIENTS

- 3 average sized avocados, halved
- 1 ib. small shrimp, precooked (40 to 50 count)
- 1 medium Roma tomato, diced very small
- ⅓ medium English cucumber, diced very small
- ⅓ cup red onion, diced very small
- ¼ cup fresh cilantro, finely minced
- 2 to 3 tbsp. lime juice
- Salt, to taste
- Black pepper, to taste
- Hot sauce, to taste.

DIRECTIONS

1. From each avocado half, scoop out about 50% of the flesh and put into a large bowl and mash with a fork. (You want to widen and somewhat hollow out the area to fill the avocado halves so there's space to add the shrimp mixture, but you don't want them totally clean).

2. Add all the other ingredients and stir to combine.

3. Taste the mixture and season with salt, pepper, lime juice, hot sauce, etc. to taste.

4. Spoon the mixture into the hollowed out avocados and serve immediately. Recipe is best fresh.

NUTRITION (per serving): Calories: 313 kcal | Fats: 17g | Carbs: 13g | Protein: 28.5g.

65. BAKED AVOCADO EGGS

 10 min

 30 min

 Entrees & Snacks

 4 Servings

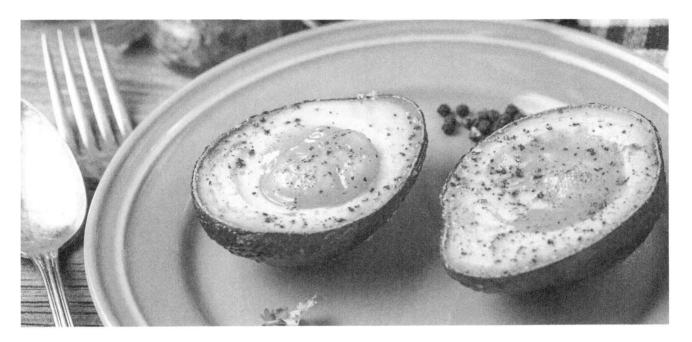

INGREDIENTS

- 2 avocados
- 4 eggs
- ½ cup bacon bits
- 2 tbsp. fresh chives, chopped
- 1 sprig of chopped fresh basil, chopped
- 1 cherry tomato, quartered
- Salt and pepper, to taste
- Cheddar cheese, shredded.

DIRECTIONS

1. Preheat the oven to 400°F.

2. Slice the avocado and remove the pits.

3. Put them on a baking sheet and crack some eggs onto the center hole of the avocado. If it's too small, just scoop out more of the flesh to make room. Salt and pepper to taste.

4. Top with bacon bits and bake for 15 minutes.

5. Remove and sprinkle with herbs. Enjoy!

NUTRITION (per serving): Calories: 271 kcal | Fats: 21g | Carbs: 6.7g | Protein: 28.1g.

66. ZUCCHINI MUFFINS

| 15 min | 15 min | Entrees & Snacks | 8 Servings |

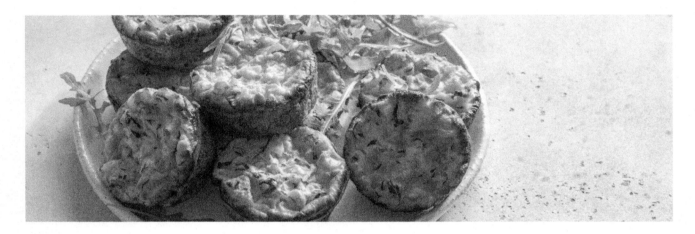

INGREDIENTS

- 4 organic eggs
- ¼ cup unsalted butter, melted
- ¼ cup water
- ⅓ cup coconut flour
- ½ tsp. organic baking powder
- ¼ tsp. salt
- 1½ cups zucchini, grated
- ½ cup Parmesan cheese, shredded
- 1 tbsp. fresh oregano, minced
- 1 tbsp. fresh thyme, minced
- ¼ cup Cheddar cheese, grated.

DIRECTIONS

1. Preheat the oven to 400°F.

2. Lightly, grease 8 muffin tins.

3. Add eggs, butter, and water in a mixing bowl and beat until well combined.

4. Add the flour, baking powder, and salt, and mix well.

5. Add remaining ingredients except for cheddar and mix until just combined.

6. Place the mixture into prepared muffin cups evenly.

7. Bake for approximately 13–15 minutes or until top of muffins become golden-brown.

8. Remove the muffin tin from oven and situate onto a wire rack for 10 minutes.

9. Carefully invert the muffins onto a platter and serve warm.

NUTRITION (per serving): Calories: 187 kcal | Fats: 23g | Carbs: 8.7g | Protein: 13.2g.

67. SAVORY VEGETABLE MUFFINS

| 15 min | 15 min | Entrees & Snacks | 12 Servings |

Breakfast Muffins are a big time saver and boost for your weight loss! Make a batch on Sunday and have them all week long. Heat them 15 seconds at a time in microwave until warm.

This version is made with roasted red pepper, Italian herbs, smoked Provolone cheese and lots of freshly grated Parmesan. You can use anything but please use a bit of shredded or chopped vegetable for a softer texture - shredded zucchini, sliced mushrooms or asparagus.

INGREDIENTS

- Vegetable cooking spray
- 8 large eggs
- ½ cup whole milk
- 1 roasted red bell pepper, from a jar, cut into fine dice
- 1 handful of fresh spinach leaves, rolled up and cut crossways into fine shreds
- ½ tsp. salt
- ¼ tsp. black pepper
- 1¼ tsp. Italian seasoning
- ½ cup Provolone cheese, shredded
- ½ cup Parmesan cheese, grated.

DIRECTIONS

1. Set oven at 375°F. Spray a 12 cups muffin tin with vegetable cooking spray, place a bit of the red pepper, spinach, and provolone into each muffin cup and set aside.

2. In a large bowl, beat the eggs and milk until smooth; add the Italian herbs, salt and pepper.

3. Using a 1/3 cup measure, scoop the mixture into the muffin tin to cover the vegetables. Fill 8 to 10 of the cups to about ¼ from the top.

4. Bake until the egg is set, tops are puffed above pan and cheese has turned golden, 12 to 15 minutes.

5. Cool for 2 minutes.

6. Generously top with the Parmesan cheese.

7. Run a butter knife around the outside of each muffin and gently remove from the tin with a large spoon.

NUTRITION (per serving): Calories: 169 kcal | Fats: 19.6g | Carbs: 11g | Protein: 9.2g.

68. MINI CRUSTLESS QUICHES

 15 min

 30 min

 Entrees & Snacks

 12 Servings

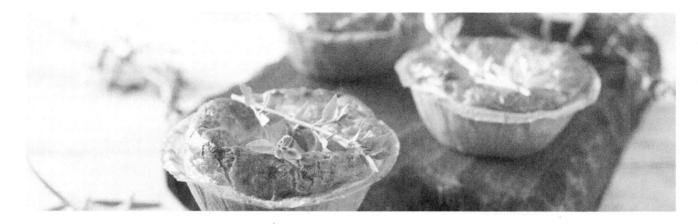

INGREDIENTS

- 1 tsp. olive oil
- 1½ cup fresh mushrooms
- 1 scallion
- 1 tsp. garlic, mince
- 1 tsp. fresh rosemary, minced
- 1 (12.3-oz.) package lite firm silken tofu
- ¼ cup unsweetened almond milk
- 2 tbsp. Parmesan cheese
- 1 tbsp. arrowroot starch
- 1 tsp. butter, softened
- ¼ tsp. ground turmeric.

DIRECTIONS

1. Set oven at 375°F. Grease a 12 cups muffin tin.

2. In a nonstick skillet, heat the oil over medium heat and sauté the scallion and garlic for about 1 minute.

3. Add the mushrooms and sauté for about 5-7 minutes.

4. Stir in the rosemary and black pepper and remove from the heat. Set aside to cool slightly.

5. In a food processor, add the tofu and remaining ingredients and pulse until smooth.

6. Transfer the tofu mixture into a large bowl.

7. Fold in the mushroom mixture. Place the mixture into the prepared muffin cups evenly. Bake for about 20-22 minutes.

8. Remove the muffin pan from the oven and place onto a wire rack to cool for about 10 minutes.

9. Carefully, invert the muffins onto wire rack and serve warm.

NUTRITION (per serving): Calories: 77 kcal | Fats: 8.7g | Carbs: 5.3g | Protein: 6.9g.

69. CALIFORNIA ROLL BITES

10 min

0 min

Entrees & Snacks

12 Servings

INGREDIENTS

- 1 English cucumber, cut into 12 ½-inch rounds
- 12 large shrimp, cleaned, cooked and cooled
- 1 large ripe avocado
- Wasabi sauce
- Sriracha sauce.

DIRECTIONS

1. Cut avocado into 12 pieces about the size of your shrimp.
2. Arrange the cucumber slices on a decorative tray, top with a shrimp, avocado piece, a dime sized drop of wasabi sauce, a squeeze of Sriracha sauce.
3. Skewer with a bamboo pick. Enjoy!

NUTRITION (per serving): Calories: 78 kcal | Fats: 2g | Carbs: 1g | Protein: 11g.

70. STUFFED CELERY CRACK

10 min

20 min

Entrees & Snacks

12 Servings

INGREDIENTS

- 1 bunch of celery
- 1 (8-oz.) block cream cheese
- 1 cup dill pickles, chopped
- 1 tbsp. dill pickles juice
- ½ tsp. salt
- 6 crispy bacon strips, chopped
- 3 tbsp. grease (or mayo)
- ¾ tsp. onion powder
- ½ tsp. parsley
- ¾ tsp. garlic powder
- ¼ tsp. dried or fresh dill.

DIRECTIONS

1. Wash the celery and cut it into about 4" pieces (or smaller, as desired).
2. Mix all ingredients below celery together well, then with a spoon begin filling each stalk very well and sprinkle with the dill.
3. Optional: add 1/2 chopped olives, 1/2 chopped pickles and without the bacon.

NUTRITION (per serving): Calories: 32 kcal | Fats: 3.3g | Carbs: 1g | Protein: 3.4g.

71. SMOKED TOFU QUESADILLAS

6 min

5 min

Entrees & Snacks

4 Servings

INGREDIENTS

- 1 lb. Extra firm sliced tofu
- 12 whole wheat tortillas
- 2 tbsp. coconut oil
- 6 slices Cheddar cheese
- 2 tbsp. Sundried tomatoes
- 1 tbsp. Cilantro
- 5 tbsp. Sour cream.

DIRECTIONS

1. Lay one tortilla flat and fill with tofu, tomato, cheese, and top with oil. Repeat for as many as you need.

2. Bake for 5 minutes and remove from flame.

3. Top with sour cream.

NUTRITION (per serving): Calories: 136 kcal | Fats: 6g | Carbs: 13g | Protein: 8g.

72. ZUCCHINI PIZZA BOATS

5 min

30 min

Entrees & Snacks

4 Servings

INGREDIENTS

- 4 medium zucchinis
- 1 cup tomato sauce
- 1 cup shredded mozzarella cheese
- 4 tbsp. Parmesan cheese.

DIRECTIONS

1. Set oven to 350°F.

2. Slice zucchini in half lengthwise and spoon out the core and seeds to form boats.

3. Place zucchini halves skin side down in a small baking dish.

4. Add remaining ingredients inside the hollow center, then set to bake until golden brown and fork tender (about 30 minutes).

5. Serve and enjoy.

NUTRITION (per serving): Calories: 214 kcal | Fats: 8g | Carbs: 24g | Protein: 6g.

Chapter 9

VEGETARIAN MAINS RECIPES

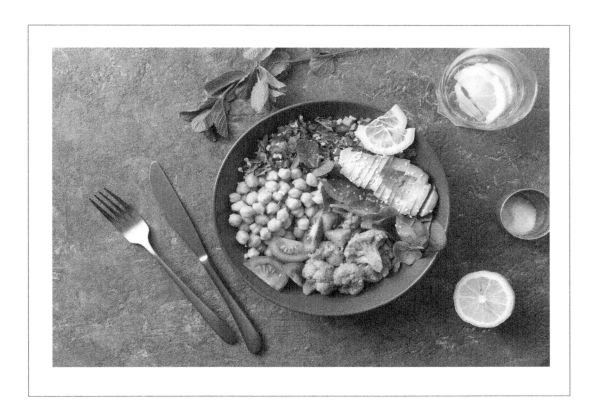

73. VEGGIE MAC BURGER

5 min   30 min   Vegetarian Mains   2 Servings

INGREDIENTS

- 1 whole wheat Burger Bun
- 1 Boca Burger, mushroom mozzarella flavor
- 2 Lettuce leaves
- 1 onion
- 1 tomato
- 1 tbsp. ketchup and mustard
- 1 tbsp. Miracle whip (light).

DIRECTIONS

1. Use the direction provided in the package of the Boca Burger.

1. After doing so, place the Boca Burger onto the buns and apply toppings such as ketchup, lettuce, onion, tomato, and miracle whip light.

2. Instead of Boca Burger, you can also use lean ground meats from beef or turkey breasts.

NUTRITION (per serving): Calories: 460 kcal | Fats: 18,6g | Carbs: 61g | Protein: 10,6g.

74. QUINOA TABBOULEH SALAD

20 min   0 min   Vegetarian Mains   4 Servings

INGREDIENTS

- 2 cups pre-cooked quinoa
- 1 medium cucumber, diced
- 1 medium tomato, diced
- ½ medium red onion, diced
- ¼ cup mint leaves, chopped
- ½ cup fresh parsley, chopped
- 1 small garlic clove, minced
- 1 tbsp. lemon juice
- 1 tbsp. extra-virgin olive oil.

DIRECTIONS

1. In a large bowl, mix all ingredients.

2. Season with salt and pepper to taste.

NUTRITION (per serving): Calories: 150 kcal | Fats: 4.5g | Carbs: 24g | Protein: 5g.

75. NO CRUST SPINACH & SWISS QUICHE

 5 min

 55 min

 Vegetarian Mains

 6 Servings

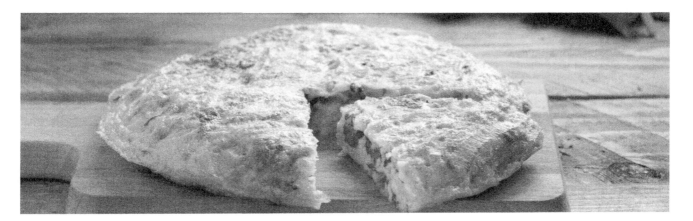

INGREDIENTS

- 1 small onion, diced
- 1 tbsp. butter
- 1 package frozen chopped spinach, thawed and squeezed dry
- 6 large eggs
- 1 cup milk
- ½ tsp. salt
- ¼ tsp. pepper
- ⅛ tsp. ground nutmeg
- 1 cup (4 oz.) Swiss cheese, grated.

DIRECTIONS

1. Preheat your oven to 325°F. Place your pie plate on a cookie sheet and lightly coat with non-stick cooking spray.

2. Sauté the onion in the butter until the onion is soft and golden. Add the spinach and sauté 2 to 3 minutes. Set aside to cool while you prepare the custard.

3. Beat eggs until well blended. Whisk in the milk, salt pepper, and nutmeg. Arrange half the cheese in the bottom of the prepared dish, add the sauteed vegetables, pour in the egg mixture to fill to the top and sprinkle with the remaining cheese.

4. Bake until just set and slightly puffed around the sides as in the photo, but still a tiny bit jiggly or soft in the two-inch circle of the center when you gently shake the oven rack. Usually, a pie will bake for about 25 minutes, but begin checking it at 20 minutes and cook until it is done.

5. Let cool for 15 minutes, cut it into wedges and serve.

NUTRITION (per serving): Calories: 310 kcal | Fats: 14g | Carbs: 26g | Protein: 10g.

76. BARLEY-MUSHROOM RISOTTO

5 min

55 min

Vegetarian Mains

6 Servings

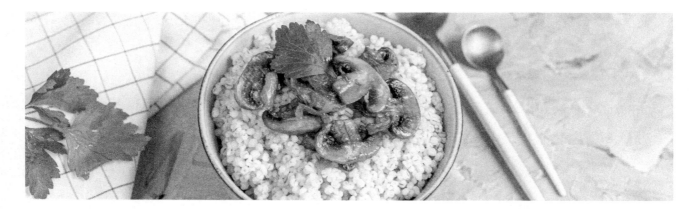

INGREDIENTS

- 1 tsp. garlic, minced
- 4 cups mushrooms, sliced
- 1 tbsp. extra-virgin olive oil
- ½ cup dry white wine
- 1 cup water
- 2 medium whole leeks, chopped
- ½ cup pearl barley
- 2 tsp. thyme, dried
- 1½ cups low sodium chicken or vegetable stock
- 3 cups fresh spinach leaves.

DIRECTIONS

1. Heat the olive oil in a large pan set over medium heat. Pour in garlic and sauté for a minute. Stir in the leeks and stir-fry for about 3 minutes or until it's soft.

2. Pour in the mushrooms and leave it to cook until it's soft and golden brown. This should take about 4 minutes.

3. Add the barley and thyme. Stir and leave it to cook for an additional 2 minutes.

4. Pour in the wine and stir gently. Lower the heat and let it simmer for a roughly 5 minutes or until all the liquid has dried up.

5. Stir in the water and stock. Leave the heat on low, put the lid on and leave it to simmer for about 40 minutes.

6. Don't forget to stir every once in a while, to ensure the barley doesn't get stuck to the bottom of the pan.

7. Now slowly add the spinach and stir until it wilts. Serve warm.

NUTRITION (per serving): Calories: 104 kcal | Fats: 3g | Carbs: 16g | Protein: 3g.

77. ROASTED VEGETABLE QUINOA SALAD WITH CHICKPEAS

15 min

30 min

Vegetarian Mains

6 Servings

INGREDIENTS

- 1 small zucchini, diced
- 1 cup low sodium chicken or vegetable stock
- 1 small eggplant, diced
- 1 tbsp. basil, dried
- 1 small yellow summer squash, diced
- 3 tbsp. extra virgin olive oil
- 1 tsp. fresh garlic, minced
- ½ cup grape tomatoes, halved
- 2 tbsp. fresh lemon juice
- 1 can chickpeas, drained and rinsed
- ⅓ cup packaged quinoa
- 1 tsp. oregano, dried.

DIRECTIONS

1. First things first, prepare your oven. Heat to 425°F.

1. Get a sheet pan ready by lining it with parchment paper.

2. Now place the zucchini, tomatoes, eggplant, chickpeas, and yellow squash on the baking sheet. Spread them out and then drizzle 1 tablespoon of olive oil into the pan. Toss to coat.

3. Slide the pan into the oven to bake for about 30 minutes. Stir only once. When it is ready, it should be soft and juicy. Not the chickpeas though, those will be crisp and firm.

4. You can do other things while the veggies roast. Place a small saucepan over medium heat and pour in stock and quinoa. Place the lid on the pan and leave it to boil. Once it is boiling, lower the heat and leave it to simmer for just 15 minutes. You should find that all the liquid has been absorbed. Turn off the heat and use a fork to fluff the quinoa. Set aside

5. Get a small bowl. Pour 1 garlic, 2 tablespoons of olive oil, and lemon juice. Mix thoroughly. Now stir in oregano and basil until thoroughly mixed.

6. To serve, mix the quinoa, veggies, and garlic dressing. Stir very gently. Enjoy!

Notes: if you would like to increase the protein content of this recipe, just serve with lean grilled chicken breast or a piece of baked fish. Feel free to scoop some low-fat plain Greek yogurt in the mixture.

NUTRITION (per serving): Calories: 200 kcal | Fats: 9g | Carbs: 27g | Protein: 7g.

78. CURRIED EGGPLANT AND CHICKPEA QUINOA

 15 min

 20 min

 Vegetarian Mains

 8 Servings

INGREDIENTS

- 1 medium red bell pepper, diced
- ¼ tsp. cayenne pepper
- 1 tsp. extra-virgin olive oil
- 2 tsp. smoked paprika
- 4 tsp. garlic, minced
- 1 large onion, chopped
- ½ cup water
- 1 tsp. turmeric powder
- 1 cup chicken and vegetable stock
- 1 medium eggplant, chopped
- 3 medium tomatoes, chopped
- Low-fat plain greek yogurt
- 1 can chickpeas, drained and rinsed
- 1 medium yellow summer squash, chopped
- ½ cup packaged quinoa.

DIRECTIONS

1. Drizzle olive oil into a large pan and place it over medium heat. Pour in garlic and stir-fry for about 1 minute.

2. Stir in bell pepper and onion, then continue to stir-fry for about 3 minutes or until soft.

3. Sprinkle turmeric, cayenne pepper, cumin, and smoked paprika. Leave to cook for 2 minutes.

4. Stir in eggplant, tomatoes, chickpeas, squash, and water. Place a lid on the pan and lower the heat just a little bit and let it cook for 15 minutes.

5. Meanwhile, as you wait for the chickpeas and veggies to cook, whip about a saucepan and place it over medium heat. In goes the stock and quinoa. Cover the saucepan and leave it to boil.

6. Once that happens, lower the heat and allow it to simmer until the quinoa absorbs all the stock. This usually takes about 15 minutes.

7. Take the saucepan off the heat and fluff the quinoa.

8. To serve, scoop some quinoa into a plate and serve with curried vegetables and a scoop of yogurt.

NUTRITION (per serving): Calories: 131 kcal | Fats: 2g | Carbs: 23g | Protein: 6g.

79. VEGAN SHEPHERD'S PIE

 15 min

 45 min

 Vegetarian Mains

 4 Servings

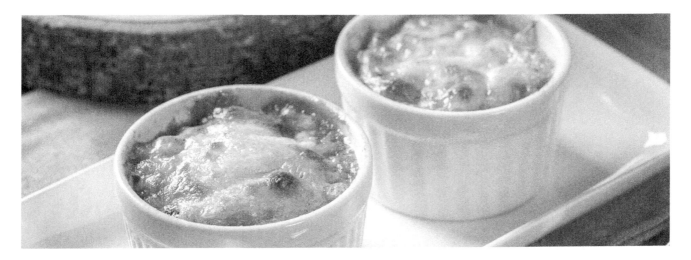

INGREDIENTS

- 1 lb. cooked potatoes, mashed
- 2 tbsp. olive oil
- 1 medium onion, chopped
- 3 garlic cloves, minced
- 1 cup cooked lentils
- 1 cup vegetable stock
- 1 tsp. thyme, dried
- 3 tbsp. fresh parsley, chopped
- 2 cups frozen mixed vegetables
- Salt and pepper to taste.

DIRECTIONS

1. Preheat oven to 425°F.

2. Coat a large skillet with olive oil.

3. Sauté onion, garlic, lentils, thyme, parsley, and frozen vegetables over medium heat for 1-2 minutes.

4. Deglaze the skillet with vegetable stock. Stir well.

5. Season vegetable mixture with salt and pepper to taste.

6. Divide the vegetable mixture evenly into 4 small ramekins, or heatproof cups.

7. Top the mixture with an even coat of 1-2 tablespoons of mashed potatoes.

8. Bake at 425°F for 15 minutes or until the mashed potatoes on top is lightly golden.

NUTRITION (per serving): Calories: 194 kcal | Fats: 2.7g | Carbs: 39g | Protein: 9g.

80. CHICKPEAS CURRY

15 min   20 min   Vegetarian Mains   8 Servings

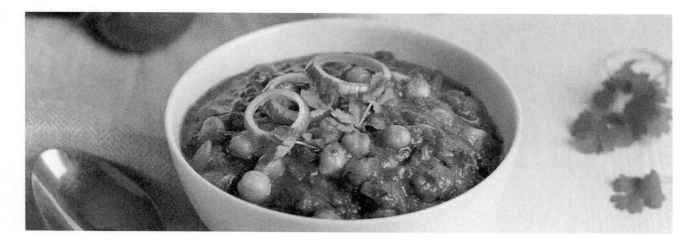

INGREDIENTS

- 1 (15 oz.) cans chickpeas, rinsed and drained
- 1 tbsp. olive oil
- 1 large onion, chopped
- 1 garlic clove, minced
- 1 tbsp. curry powder
- 1 cup vegetable stock
- ¼ cup cilantro, freshly chopped
- Salt and pepper, to taste.

DIRECTIONS

1. In a cooking pan, heat the olive oil over medium heat. Add chopped onion. Stir until the onion is softened and starting to brown.

2. Slightly reduce the heat, add garlic, stir for 30 seconds or until fragrant.

3. Stir in the curry powder, cook for additional 30 seconds.

4. Add drained chickpeas and vegetable stock to the pan. Continue to cook and stir all ingredients together.

5. Bring to a boil, reduce the heat, and let it continue to simmer for about 10-15 minutes.

6. Add salt and paper to taste.

7. Turn off the heat and garnish the chickpeas curry with freshly chopped cilantro.

NUTRITION (per serving): Calories: 177 kcal | Fats: 3g | Carbs: 32g | Protein: 9g.

81. MEXICAN STUFFED SUMMER SQUASH

15 min

30 min

Vegetarian Mains

6 Servings

INGREDIENTS

- 1 medium yellow summer squash
- ½ cup quinoa, cooked
- 1 small tomato, diced
- ½ cup refried black beans
- ¼ cup Colby jack cheese, grated
- 2 small scallions, chopped
- 2 tbsp. black olives, chopped
- Nonstick cooking spray.

DIRECTIONS

1. Prepare your oven. Preheat to 400°F.

2. Grease an 8-by-8-inch baking dish with enough cooking spray.

3. Remove and dispose of the ends of the summer squash. Slice it in half horizontally and then remove and dispose of the seeds with a spoon.

4. Now put the squash on a greased baking dish with the cut side down.

5. Use something small to create holes in the squash so that it can breathe. Now pour a tablespoon of water into the dish.

6. Place the baking dish in the microwave and leave it to heat for 3 minutes or until it feels soft. Bring it out and drain any excess water.

7. Leave the squash to cool until it is cold enough to touch.

8. Now place the squash so that the cut sides are facing up and far away from each other

9. Scoop ¼ cup of beans into each squash and then layer ¼ cup of quinoa. Pour Colby jack cheese over the top and cover the dish with foil.

10. Slide the dish into the oven to bake for about 25 minutes.

11. When 25 minutes is up, take out the foil and bake for another 5 minutes or until you see the cheese looking all bubbly.

12. For garnishing, top with olives, scallions, and tomatoes right before you serve.

NUTRITION (per serving): Calories: 190 kcal | Fats: 8g | Carbs: 21g | Protein: 9g.

82. COCONUT CURRY TOFU BOWL

 45 min   30 min   Vegetarian Mains   6 Servings

INGREDIENTS

- 1 tbsp. ginger, grated
- 1 package extra-firm tofu
- 1 medium jalapeño pepper, finely chopped seeded
- 2 tbsp. curry powder
- 3 tsp. coconut oil
- 1 medium yellow bell pepper, chopped
- 4 tsp. garlic, minced
- 2 mediums carrots, chopped
- ½ tsp. cumin powder
- 2 cups coconut milk, unflavored and unsweetened
- 1 medium bok choy, with the leaves and stems chopped
- ⅛ tsp. cinnamon powder
- 4 oz. canned tomato sauce
- Cauliflower rice
- ½ cup low sodium chicken or vegetable stock)
- ¼ cup cilantro, finely chopped.

DIRECTIONS

1. Remove excess water from the tofu and place it in a bowl lined with paper towels. Place some extra layers of paper towel on top of the tofu. If you don't have extra paper towels, use a clean dish towel.
2. Place a heavy skillet on top of the paper towel or dish towel for extra weight. Leave that set up alone for about 30 minutes to drain as much water as possible.
3. Now transfer the tofu to a clean chopping board and slice it in half horizontally, then dice it into 1-by-2-inch pieces. Set aside.
4. Place a large skillet over medium heat and drizzle 1 ½ teaspoon of coconut oil into it. As soon as the oil is hot and steaming, gently drop the tofu cubes into it to cook for about 15 minutes or until it looks golden brown on both sides. When it's ready, pour the tofu cubes into a dish and set aside.
5. Drizzle the leftover coconut oil, about 1 ½ teaspoon into the same pan used to fry the tofu. When the oil is hot and steaming, gently pour in ginger, bell pepper, bok choy stems, jalapeño, garlic, and carrots. Gently stir fry for 10 minutes or extra if the veggies are not tender enough.
6. Sprinkle turmeric powder, cinnamon powder, curry powder, and cumin powder. Stir thoroughly.
7. The next thing to do is add tomato sauce, stock, and coconut milk. Stir thoroughly
8. Add bok choy leaves and tofu, then fold them in. Leave this to simmer for about 10 minutes or more if the leaves haven't wilted.
9. To serve, scoop some cauliflower rice into a bowl, then top with tofu sauce. For garnishing, use cilantro.

NUTRITION (per serving): Calories: 219 kcal | Fats: 8g | Carbs: 21g | Protein: 15g.

83. BAKED EGGPLANT

10 min

50 min

Vegetarian Mains

4 Servings

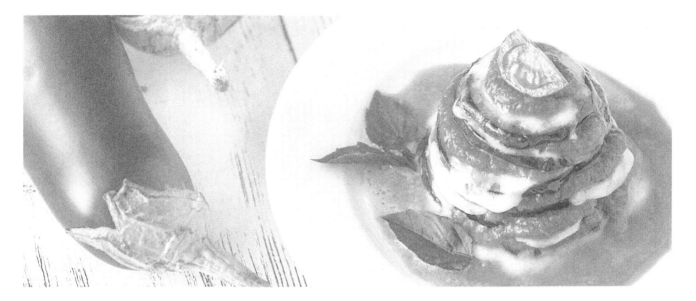

INGREDIENTS

- 1 medium eggplant, peeled and sliced
- 3 to 4 tbsp. olive oil
- ½ cup Parmesan cheese, grated
- ½ cup part-skim Mozzarella cheese, shredded
- ½ cup fresh flat leaf parsley, finely chopped
- Sea salt and freshly ground black pepper
- 2 cups marinara sauce.

DIRECTIONS

1. Preheat oven to 400°F.

2. Arrange eggplant slices on a baking sheet that has been lightly sprayed with nonstick vegetable cooking spray.

3. Drizzle each slice with a little olive oil, season with salt and bake until lightly browned and tender, 20 to 25 minutes, turning halfway through. Remove to cool.

4. Arrange the eggplant in an even layer in small square baking dish - spread with sauce, sprinkle with parmesan and mozzarella and repeat with additional layers.

5. Bake until bubbling and golden, 20 to 25 minutes.

6. Cool 10 minutes before serving.

NUTRITION (per serving): Calories: 49.6 kcal | Fats: 1.4g | Carbs: 9.4g | Protein: 0.2g.

84. ZUCCHINI LASAGNA ROLL-UPS

 30 min

 30 min

 Vegetarian Mains

6 Servings

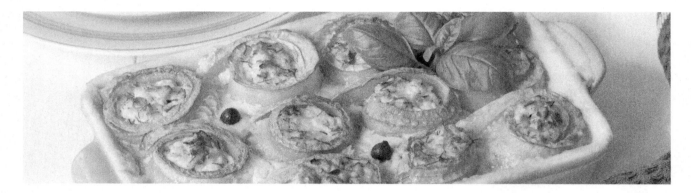

INGREDIENTS

- 3 large zucchini, trimmed and sliced lengthwise into -inch-thick strips
- 1 tsp. salt
- Nonstick cooking spray
- 1 (10-ounce) bag fresh spinach
- 1 cup part-skim ricotta
- ½ cup Parmesan cheese
- 1 large egg
- 2 garlic cloves, minced
- 2 tsp. Italian seasoning
- 1½ cups marinara sauce
- 1 cup part-skim Mozzarella, shredded.

DIRECTIONS

1. Preheat the oven to 400°F.
2. Lay the zucchini slices flat on a paper towel-lined baking sheet, and sprinkle with salt. Let sit for 15 minutes.
3. Meanwhile, spray a small skillet with nonstick cooking spray, and set over medium heat. Add the spinach and cook for 2 minutes, or until wilted. Remove from the heat.
4. In a medium bowl, mix the ricotta, Parmesan, egg, garlic, and Italian seasoning until well combined.
5. Pat the zucchini dry, removing excess salt.
6. Spread 1 cup of marinara in the bottom of a 9-by-9-inch baking dish. Spread each zucchini slice with a spoonful of ricotta mixture, then gently roll up and place in the prepared baking dish, seam-side down. Repeat with the remaining zucchini and filling. Top with the remaining ½ cup of marinara, and sprinkle with the mozzarella cheese.
7. Bake for 25 to 30 minutes, or until the lasagna rolls are heated through, and the cheese begins to brown.
8. Serve immediately.

NUTRITION (per serving): Calories: 240 kcal | Fats: 13g | Carbs: 16g | Protein: 18g.

85. TOFU STIR-FRY

| 15 min | 40 min | Vegetarian Mains | 4 Servings |

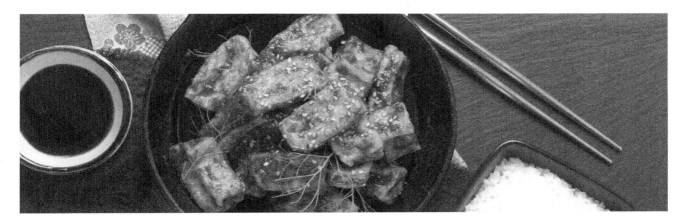

INGREDIENTS

- 1 (14-ounces) block extra-firm tofu
- Nonstick cooking spray
- 1 tbsp. sesame oil
- 3 cups frozen stir-fry vegetable blend
- ½ cup Stir-Fry Sauce.

DIRECTIONS

1. Drain the tofu and wrap in a kitchen towel. Place a plate on top of the tofu, and top with something heavy, such as a book or skillet. Let dry for 15 minutes, changing the towel if necessary.

2. Once dry, chop into 1-inch cubes or rectangles. Arrange the tofu on a lightly greased or parchment paper-covered baking sheet, and bake for 25 to 35 minutes, or until golden brown, flipping halfway through. Once golden brown, remove from the oven and let cool while you continue cooking.

3. Heat a large skillet over medium-high heat. Add the sesame oil and swirl to coat. Add the veggies and stir-fry or toss to coat. Cook for 5 minutes.

4. Add the stir-fry sauce and stir to coat. Add the tofu and stir. Cook for 3 to 5 minutes, gently stirring constantly.

5. When the veggies reach the tenderness of your liking, remove from the heat, and serve.

NUTRITION (per serving): Calories: 163 kcal | Fats: 8g | Carbs: 11g | Protein: 12g.

86. SPAGHETTI SQUASH CHOW MEIN

10 min

55 min

Vegetarian Mains

3 Servings

A healthier low-carb version of everyone's favorite takeout dish.
Even your picky eaters will love this!
Only 252 kcal/serving!

INGREDIENTS

- Nonstick cooking spray
- 1 small (3-to 4-pound) spaghetti squash
- ¼ cup low-sodium soy sauce
- 3 garlic cloves, minced
- 1 tbsp. oyster sauce
- 1 inch ginger root, peeled and minced
- 2 tbsp. extra-virgin olive oil
- 1 small white onion, diced
- 3 celery stalks, thinly sliced
- 2 cups shredded cabbage (or coleslaw mix).

DIRECTIONS

1. Preheat the oven to 350°F. Coat a baking sheet with cooking spray.

2. Halve the spaghetti squash, remove and discard the seeds, and place the halves cut side down on the prepared baking sheet. Bake for 30 to 45 minutes, or until the flesh is tender and can be scraped with a fork.

3. Remove from the oven and let cool. Scrape out the flesh with a fork, creating small noodles. Set aside.

4. In a small bowl, whisk together the soy sauce, garlic, oyster sauce, and ginger.

5. In a large skillet over medium heat, heat the oil. Add the onion and celery and cook, stirring, until tender, 3 to 4 minutes.

6. Add the cabbage and cook, stirring, until heated through, 1 to 2 minutes.

7. Add the spaghetti squash and sauce mixture. Continue cooking for another 2 minutes.

8. Serve immediately.

NUTRITION (per serving): Calories: 252 kcal | Fats: 11g | Carbs: 39g | Protein: 6g.

Chapter 10

FISH & SEAFOOD MAINS RECIPES

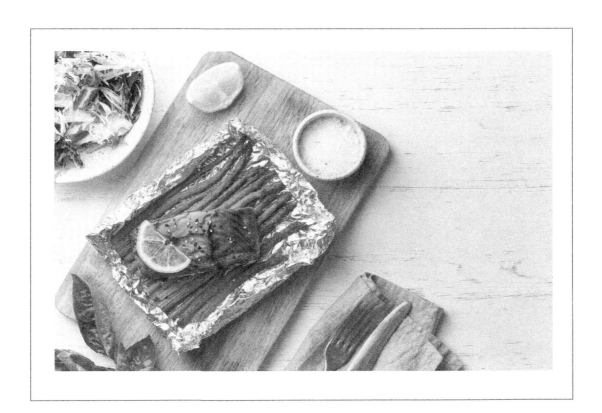

87. FISH TACO SALAD

10 min

10 min

Fish & Seafood Mains

4 Servings

This fish taco salad is a healthier version of fish tacos, that is so filling and full of flavor, you won't even miss the tortillas! You'll never know you're doing your body good while you're enjoying this healthy, delicious Fish Taco Salad!

INGREDIENTS

For the Fish:

- 1½ pounds wild-caught cod
- 1 tbsp. extra-virgin olive oil
- 2 tbsp. Taco Seasoning
- Salt, to taste
- Freshly ground black pepper, to taste

For the Salad:

- 8 cups lettuce, shredded
- 2 cups cauliflower rice, steamed
- ½ cup black beans
- 1 red bell pepper, diced
- 1 avocado, peeled and diced
- ½ cup pico de gallo
- 1 lime, quartered.

DIRECTIONS

1. Cut the fish into 4 equal-size portions.

2. In a large bowl, combine the fish, olive oil, and taco seasoning, and gently toss to coat.

3. Heat a grill or skillet over medium heat. When hot, add the fish and cook until it is brown and flakes easily, about 3 minutes per side. Season with salt and pepper as desired.

4. Divide the shredded lettuce, cauliflower rice, black beans, bell pepper, avocado, and fish evenly among 4 plates.

5. Dress with the pico de gallo and lime wedges for squeezing and serve.

NUTRITION (per serving): Calories: 328 kcal | Fats: 11g | Carbs: 23g | Protein: 36g.

88. HALIBUT WITH CREAMY PARMESAN-DILL SAUCE

5 min

20 min

Fish & Seafood Mains

4 Servings

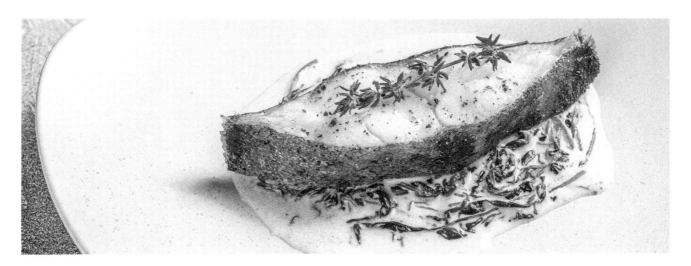

INGREDIENTS

- 4 (6-ounce) fresh halibut fillets (1-inch thick)
- ½ lemon juice
- Salt and black pepper, to taste
- ⅓ cup low-fat sour cream
- ⅓ cup low-fat, plain Greek yogurt
- ⅓ cup Parmesan cheese
- ½ tsp. garlic powder
- ½ tsp. dried dill
- 3 scallions, finely chopped.

DIRECTIONS

1. Preheat the oven to 400°F.
2. Place the halibut fillets in a large baking dish and add the lemon juice. Season with salt and pepper to taste.
3. In a small bowl, mix the sour cream, yogurt, cheese, garlic powder, dill, and scallions. Spread the mixture over the fish.
4. Bake for 15 to 20 minutes, or until the internal temperature reaches 145°F, the fish is opaque and flakes easily with a fork, and the cheese is golden.
5. Serve hot and engoy!

NUTRITION (per serving): Calories: 345 kcal | Fats: 12g | Carbs: 6g | Protein: 52g.

89. BLACKENED SALMON WITH AVOCADO CREAM

 10 min

 10 min

 Fish & Seafood Mains

 4 Servings

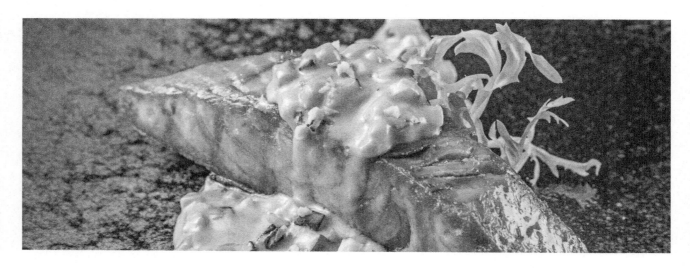

INGREDIENTS

- 4 (6-ounce) salmon fillets, bones removed
- 1 tbsp. butter, melted
- 2 tbsp. blackened seasoning
- 1 tbsp. extra-virgin olive oil
- ½ cup Avocado Cream.

DIRECTIONS

1. Pat the salmon fillets dry on both sides with paper towels.

2. Brush the butter over the fleshy side of the salmon fillets.

3. Pour the seasoning onto a plate and press the flesh side of each salmon fillet into the seasoning, coating evenly.

4. In a large skillet over medium heat, heat the olive oil. Add the salmon, skin-side up, and cook until blackened, 3 to 4 minutes.

5. Flip the fillets and continue to cook to your liking, 5 to 7 minutes, depending on the thickness of the fillets, or to an internal temperature of 125 to 145°F. Once done, the fish should flake easily with a fork.

6. Transfer to individual plates, and serve with the avocado cream.

NUTRITION (per serving): Calories: 356kcal | Fats: 24g | Carbs: 2g | Protein: 35g.

90. MEDITERRANEAN BAKED FISH WITH TOMATOES OLIVES & CAPERS

5 min

30 min

Fish & Seafood Mains

6 Servings

INGREDIENTS

- ⅓ cup extra-virgin olive oil
- 1 small red onion, finely chopped
- 1 cup grape tomatoes, cut into quarters
- 5 garlic cloves, chopped
- 1½ tsp. ground coriander
- 1 tsp. sweet Spanish paprika
- 1 tsp. ground cumin
- ½ tsp. cayenne pepper (optional)
- ½ cup sliced pitted Kalamata olives
- 1½ tbsp. capers
- Salt and pepper
- 1½ lb white fish fillet, such as cod fillet or halibut fillet
- ½ lemon fresh juice
- Zest of 1 lemon
- Fresh parsley or mint for garnish.

DIRECTIONS

1. Prepare the sauce: In a medium saucepan, heat extra virgin olive oil over medium-high heat until shimmering but not smoking. Add onions, cook for 3 minutes until it begins to turn gold in color, tossing regularly. Add tomatoes, garlic, spices, pinch of salt (not too much), pepper, capers, and olives. Bring to a boil, then turn heat down to medium-low and let simmer for 15 minutes or so.

2. Heat oven to 400°F.

3. Pat fish dry and season with salt and pepper on both sides.

4. Pour ½ of the cooked tomato sauce into the bottom of a 9x13-inch baking dish. Arrange the fish on top. Add lemon juice and lemon zest, then top with the remaining tomato sauce.

5. Bake in 400°F heated oven for 15 to 18 minutes or until fish is cooked through and flakes easily (do not over-cook). Remove from heat and garnish with fresh parsley or mint to your liking.

6. Serve hot and enjoy!

NUTRITION (per serving): Calories: 308 kcal | Fats: 17.4g | Carbs: 13.3g | Protein: 27g.

91. TUNA PATTIES

5 min

20 min

Fish & Seafood Mains

8 Servings

INGREDIENTS

- 4 (3-ounces) tuna cans
- 16 cracker pieces, crushed
- 4 egg whites
- ¼ cup carrot, grated
- 1 tbsp. onion, finely sliced
- Dried mustard
- Ground pepper, to taste
- ¼ cup water chestnuts (sliced red peppers or capers will do), chopped.

DIRECTIONS

1. Prepare a bowl and mix all the ingredients in one go.
2. Blend them thoroughly using your hands.
3. Form patties. With the ingredients provided above, you can form about 8 patties.
4. Use nonstick cooking spray onto a medium-sized skillet.
5. Heat the skillet over medium temperature.
6. Cook the patties for about 2 to 3 minutes, or until it's golden brown consistency on each side is achieved.

NUTRITION (per serving): Calories: 130 kcal | Fats: 4,9g | Carbs: 0,3g | Protein: 15,8g.

92. SHRIMP CEVICHE

10 min

30 min

Fish & Seafood Mains

4 Servings

INGREDIENTS

- 1 lb. cooked jumbo shrimp
- 1 cup diced tomatoes
- ½ cup finely chopped red onion
- 1 jalapeño pepper, minced
- ¼ cup lemon and lime juice
- ½ cup chopped fresh cilantro
- Salt, to taste
- 1 avocado, pitted and peeled.

DIRECTIONS

1. In a large bowl, mix the shrimp, tomatoes, red onion, and jalapeño.
2. Pour in the lemon and lime juice, cilantro, and salt to taste. Gently toss to coat.
3. For best flavor, cover and refrigerate for at least 30 minutes.
4. Dice the avocado into half-inch chunks right before serving. Add it to the shrimps.

NUTRITION (per serving): Calories: 207 kcal | Fats: 8g | Carbs: 11g | Protein: 25g.

93. PAN-FRIED RAINBOW TROUT

 20 min

 10 min

 Fish & Seafood Mains

 2 Servings

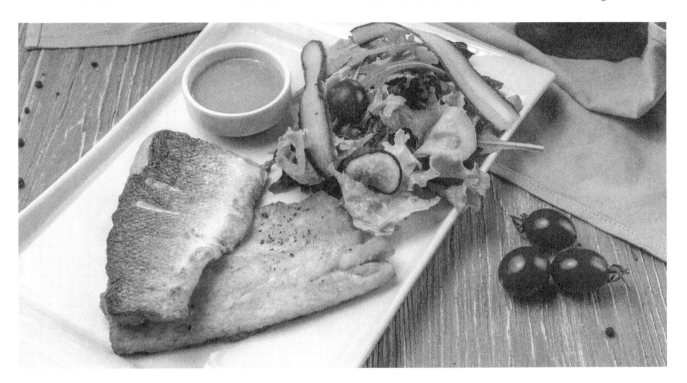

INGREDIENTS

- 8 oz. rainbow trout fillet
- 3 tbsp. yellow cornmeal
- 1⅓ tbsp. parsley, chopped
- ¼ tsp. ground celery seeds
- ¼ tsp ground black pepper
- 1 pinch salt
- 2 tsp olive oil.

DIRECTIONS

1. Clean and rinse fish fillets. Check to make sure all bones are removed. Pat dry.

2. Mix together cornmeal, salt, pepper, celery seed and chopped parsley.

3. Cover fish with cornmeal mixture and press onto fish.

4. Heat olive oil in non-stick skillet. Cook fish 2 to 3 minutes per side. Fish should be brown and crisp and should flake when pierced with a fork.

NUTRITION (per serving): Calories: 240 kcal | Fats: 10g | Carbs: 10g | Protein: 25g.

94. SOY-GINGER SALMON WITH BOK CHOY

20 min

10 min

Fish & Seafood Mains

4 Servings

INGREDIENTS

- ¼ cup low-sodium soy sauce
- 2 tsp. rice vinegar
- 1 tbsp. brown sugar
- 2 tsp. grated ginger
- 2 garlic cloves, minced
- 2 scallions, chopped
- 1 lb. wild-caught Alaskan salmon fillet, cut into 4 pieces, bones removed
- 4 baby bok choy, quartered lengthwise
- 2 tsp. extra-virgin olive oil
- Salt
- Freshly ground black pepper.

DIRECTIONS

1. In a resealable bag, combine the soy sauce, vinegar, brown sugar, ginger, garlic, and scallions.

2. Add the salmon and mix to coat. Chill for 15 to 30 minutes.

3. Preheat the oven to 400°F. Line a baking sheet with aluminum foil.

4. Remove the salmon from the bag, reserving any marinade, and place the salmon skin-side down on one side of the baking sheet.

5. Place the bok choy on the other side of the baking sheet, drizzle on the olive oil, and toss to coat. Season with salt and pepper to taste.

6. Bake for 10 to 12 minutes, or until the internal temperature of the salmon reaches 125 to 145°F, and the bok choy is tender.

7. Meanwhile, in a small saucepan, heat the reserved marinade to a boil. Simmer on low until thickened and reduced by half, 5 to 10 minutes.

8. Transfer the salmon and bok choy to four plates, cover the salmon with the warm marinade and serve.

NUTRITION (per serving): Calories: 247 kcal | Fats: 12g | Carbs: 8g | Protein: 27g.

95. TUNA CHILI

15 min

30 min

Fish & Seafood Mains

4 Servings

INGREDIENTS

- 1 tbsp. olive oil
- 1 medium onion, chopped
- 1 can tuna (7 oz) in water, drained
- ½ can gluten- free beans (7 oz), drained
- ½ can tomatoes (7 oz), chopped
- 1 tsp. dried chili flakes
- ½ cilantro bunch, chopped
- Salt and pepper to taste.

DIRECTIONS

1. Heat 1 tablespoon of olive oil in a medium pot. Add onion and cook over medium-low heat until soft.
2. Add drained tuna, tomatoes, beans and chili flakes.
3. Cover the pot and simmer for about 15 minutes or until the tomatoes soften.
4. Season with salt and pepper.
5. Serve with chopped cilantro as garnish.

NUTRITION (per serving): Calories: 240.2 kcal | Fats: 4.3g | Carbs: 9.5g | Protein: 23.4g.

96. PAN SEARED SCALLOPS

5 min

2 min

Fish & Seafood Mains

4 Servings

INGREDIENTS

- 12 oz. fresh sea scallops
- 1 tbsp. olive oil
- Salt and pepper to taste.

DIRECTIONS

1. Rinse and pat dry the scallops. Season with salt and pepper.
2. In a large skillet, heat olive oil over medium-high heat.
3. Gently place each scallop on the heated skillet. Sear for about 1½- 2 minutes on each side (depending on the size of the scallops).

NUTRITION (per serving): Calories: 150.7 kcal | Fats: 3.4g | Carbs: 9g | Protein: 22.5g.

97. PAN SEARED COD FILLET

15 min

10 min

Fish & Seafood Mains

2 Servings

INGREDIENTS

- 2 (3 oz.) Atlantic Cod fillets
- 1 tbsp. olive oil
- 1 garlic clove, minced
- 2 lemon wedges
- 1 branch fresh thyme
- 1 branch fresh rosemary
- Salt and black pepper.

DIRECTIONS

1. Season fillets with minced garlic, a pinch of salt and black pepper. (Optional: sprinkle thyme and rosemary leaves).

2. In a preheated skillet, add 1 tablespoon of olive oil.

3. Place the fish fillets and let it cook for about 2-3 minutes on each side or until fully cooked in the center.

4. Remove fish from heat and serve with lemon wedges if desired.

NUTRITION (per serving): Calories: 90 kcal | Fats: 1g | Carbs: 2g | Protein: 19g.

98. SHRIMPS WITH TOMATO & FENNEL

5 min

25 min

Fish & Seafood Mains

4 Servings

INGREDIENTS

- 1 lb. shrimps, peeled & cleaned
- 1 cup fennel, diced
- 1 medium onion, chopped
- 2 garlic cloves, minced
- 1 tbsp. olive oil
- 1 tbsp. tomato paste
- 1 cup white wine (or broth)
- 1 cup tomatoes, crushed
- Red pepper flakes to taste
- Salt and black pepper
- 4 or 5 fresh basil leaves, minced

DIRECTIONS

1. Sauté fennel, onion, and garlic in olive oil until softened and golden.

2. Stir in tomato paste, add white wine, tomatoes, salt, pepper and a big pinch of crushed red pepper flakes to taste.

3. Bring to a boil, lower heat and allow to reduce for 15 minutes until thickened.

4. Add shrimp and poach until just cooked through. Stir in basil.

5. Serve in a deep bowl with lots of sauce.

NUTRITION (per serving): Calories: 196 kcal | Fats: 8g | Carbs: 5g | Protein: 22g.

99. SHRIMP WITH ZUCCHINI NOODLES

20 min

15 min

Fish & Seafood Mains

4 Servings

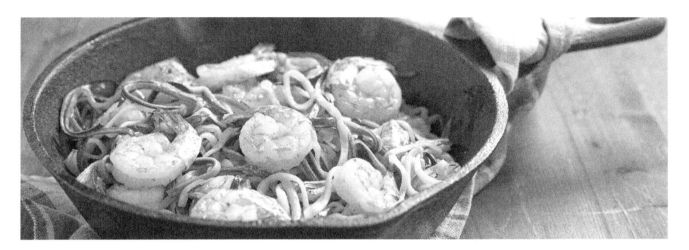

INGREDIENTS

- 4 garlic cloves, sliced
- 2 tbsp. olive oil
- ½ lemon juice
- ½ cup white wine (or chicken broth)
- ¼ tsp. red pepper, crushed
- 1 tsp. Tuscan seasoning or Italian seasoning, to taste
- Sea salt and black pepper
- 1 lb. medium shrimp, peeled and cleaned
- 2 medium zucchini.

DIRECTIONS

1. Cut zucchini using a spiralizer or gadget into long spaghetti type noodles, pat with paper towels to remove liquid and set aside (do this just before cooking).

2. Cook the garlic in the olive oil in a deep wok or skillet over medium high heat until toasted and golden, 2 to 3 minutes. Remove to a medium bowl and set aside.

3. Turn heat to high, add the shrimp and toss until just turning pink, 1 to 2 minutes. Remove to bowl with the garlic.

4. Add the lemon juice, wine, crushed red pepper, Tuscan seasoning, ½ teaspoon salt, lots of freshly ground black pepper to the hot pan and boil until slightly thickened and reduced, 3 to 4 minutes.

5. Add the zucchini pasta and toss until well coated and softened, 1 to 2 minutes.

6. Add the shrimp, garlic chips and give a final toss to combine.

NUTRITION (per serving): Calories: 240 kcal | Fats: 8g | Carbs: 11g | Protein: 32g.

100. BAKED SALMON

5 min

20 min

Fish & Seafood Mains

4 Servings

Salmon, whether fillet or steak, is an ideal fish to bake. It is a healthy, meaty fish that is full of flavor.

The skin on both cuts helps keep the flesh together while it is cooking, so make sure you buy salmon with the skin intact.

Although a good piece of salmon is delicious drizzled with just a bit of olive oil and a little salt, these recipes take that pleasant taste to a whole new level.

INGREDIENTS

- 4 (6-ounce) salmon fillets, bones removed
- ¼ cup pineapple juice
- ¼ tsp. cinnamon
- 2 tbsp. natural lemon juice
- 2 tsp. lemon rind, grated
- 2 tsp. brown sugar
  ½ tsp. salt.
- 4 tsp. chilli powder
- ¾ tsp. ground cumin.

DIRECTIONS

1. Heat the oven over 400°F.

2. Using a Ziploc bag, put Salmon fillets, lemon juice, and pineapple juice inside. Marinate for one hour in a refrigerator.

3. After an hour, remove salmon and separate the marinade.

4. Next, apply the remaining ingredients to the fish and rub.

5. Prepare a baking dish and spray with cooking oil spray. And then put the salmon fillets on it.

6. Bake for about 10 to 15 minutes or until preferred texture is achieved.

7. Lastly, garnish the salmon fillet with lemon slice

NUTRITION (per serving): Calories: 185kcal | Fats: 6g | Carbs: 0g | Protein: 28g.

Chapter 11

POULTRY MAINS RECIPES

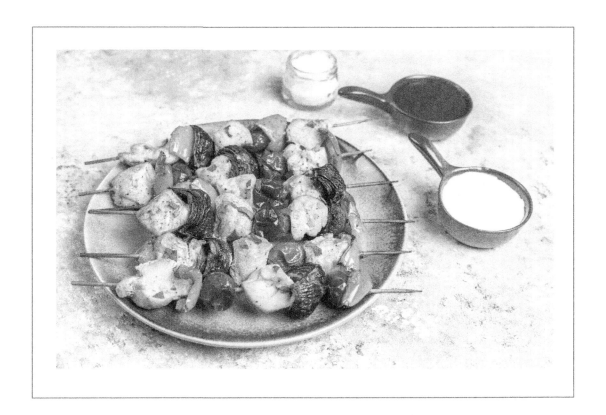

101. CREAMY CHICKEN SOUP WITH CAULIFLOWER

15 min

40 min

Poultry Mains

2 Servings

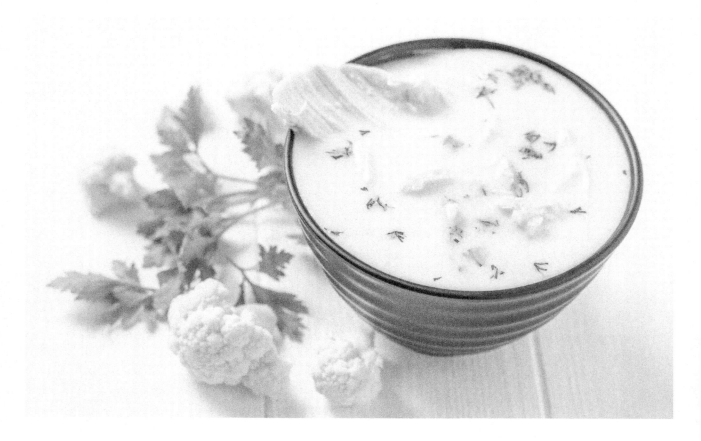

INGREDIENTS

- 1 tsp. garlic, minced
- 1 tsp. extra-virgin olive oil
- ½ yellow onion, diced
- 1 carrot, diced
- 1 celery stalk, diced
- 1½ lb. (3 or 4 medium) cooked chicken breast, diced

DIRECTIONS

1. Place a large soup pot over medium-high heat. Sauté the garlic in the olive oil for 1 minute.

2. Add the onion, carrot, and celery and sauté until tender, 3 to 5 minutes.

3. Add the chicken breast, broth, water, black pepper, thyme, and cauliflower. Bring to a simmer, reduce the heat to medium-low,

- 2 cups low-sodium chicken broth
- 2 cups water
- 1 tsp. black pepper
- 1 tsp. thyme, dried
- 2½ cups fresh cauliflower florets
- 1 cup fresh spinach, chopped
- 2 cups nonfat or 1% milk.

and cook, uncovered, for 30 minutes.

4. Add the fresh spinach and stir until wilted, about 5 minutes.

5. Stir in the milk, then serve immediately.

NUTRITION (per serving): Calories: 164 kcal | Fats: 3g | Carbs: 5g | Protein: 25g.

102. CHICKEN & BARLEY SOUP

15 min

50 min

Poultry Mains

8 Servings

INGREDIENTS

- 1 tbsp. extra-virgin olive oil
- 1 tsp. garlic, minced
- 1 large onion, diced
- 2 large carrots, chopped
- 3 celery stalks, chopped
- 1 (14.5 oz.) can diced tomatoes
- ¾ cup pearl barley
- 2½ cup diced cooked chicken
- 4 cups low-sodium chicken broth
- 2 cups water
- ½ tsp. thyme, dried
- ½ tsp. dried sage
- ¼ tsp. rosemary, dried
- 2 bay leaves.

DIRECTIONS

1. Place a large soup pot over medium-high heat. Sauté the olive oil and garlic for 1 minute.

2. Add the onion, carrots, and celery and sauté until tender, 3 to 5 minutes.

3. Add the tomatoes, barley, chicken broth, water, thyme, sage, rosemary, and bay leaves. Bring to a simmer, then reduce the heat to medium-low and cook, uncovered, for about 45 minutes. The soup is done when the barley is tender.

4. Remove and discard bay leaves before serving.

NUTRITION (per serving): Calories: 198 kcal | Fats: 3g | Carbs: 9g | Protein: 16g.

103. CHICKEN & BEAN SOUP

 5 min

 35 min

 Poultry Mains

 6 Servings

Lots of great flavors pulled from the shelves and quickly combined in this stew. This makes plenty for a supper plus either lunches or freeze for another meal!

INGREDIENTS

- 1 sweet onion, diced
- 2 garlic cloves, finely chopped
- 1 tbsp. olive oil
- 1¼ lb. chicken thighs, boneless and skinless, each cut into 4 pieces
- 1 tbsp. smoked sweet paprika
- Sea salt and black pepper, to taste
- 1 cup chicken broth
- 1 (15-ounce) can diced (fire roasted) tomatoes
- 1 (6-ounce) jar roasted red peppers, sliced
- 1 (15-ounce) can pinto beans, drained and rinsed
- 1 (5-ounce) jar marinated artichoke quarters, drained
- ¼ cup green olives with pimento
- Chopped flat leaf parsley.

DIRECTIONS

1. Sauté the onion and garlic in the olive oil over medium high heat in a heavy large, covered skillet until softened, 2 to 4 minutes.

2. Season the chicken with half of the paprika, salt and pepper and add to the pan with the onions.

3. Cook until browned, 4 to 6 minutes.

4. Stir in the rest of the paprika and then add the broth, tomatoes, roasted peppers, beans and artichokes.

5. Reduce heat cover and simmer 20 to 25 minutes, until chicken is tender.

6. Stir in the olives and parsley.

NUTRITION (per serving): Calories: 172 kcal | Fats: 4g | Carbs: 10g | Protein: 24g.

104. TURKEY MEATBALLS SOUP

30 min

35 min

Poultry Mains

8 Servings

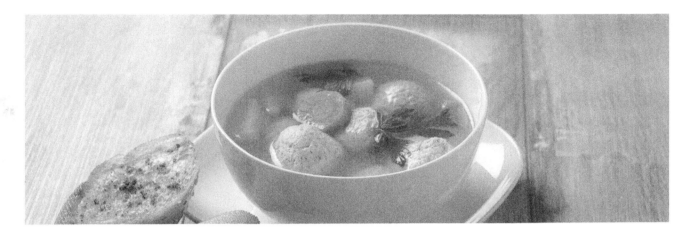

INGREDIENTS

FOR TURKEY MEATBALLS
- 1 lb. lean ground turkey
- 1 egg
- ½ cup grated Parmesan cheese
- 2 tbsp. fresh basil, chopped
- 2 garlic cloves, minced
- ¾ tsp. salt
- ¼ tsp. ground black pepper

FOR BROTH
- 8 cups low-sodium chicken broth
- 1 cup carrots, peeled and sliced
- 1 cup celery, sliced
- ¼ bunch parsley leaves, chopped
- ½ medium onion, chopped.

DIRECTIONS

1. Combine egg, turkey, Parmesan cheese, garlic, basil, salt and pepper in medium sized bowl.

2. Shape the turkey mixture by hand into meatballs. Place shaped meatballs on baking sheet or plate. Let them chill for 30 minutes.

3. While waiting for the meatballs to chill, bring chicken broth to boil, add carrots, celery, and onions. Reduce the heat and let it simmer semi- uncovered for 10 minutes.

4. Add the chilled turkey meatballs. Simmer for another 10-15 minutes. Make sure the meatballs are cooked thoroughly.

5. Stir in the parsley leaves.

6. Season with salt and pepper to taste.

NUTRITION (per serving): Calories: 169 kcal | Fats: 4.8g | Carbs: 12.6g | Protein: 17.9g.

105. CHICKEN LETTUCE WRAPS

 5 min

 20 min

 Poultry Mains

 4 Servings

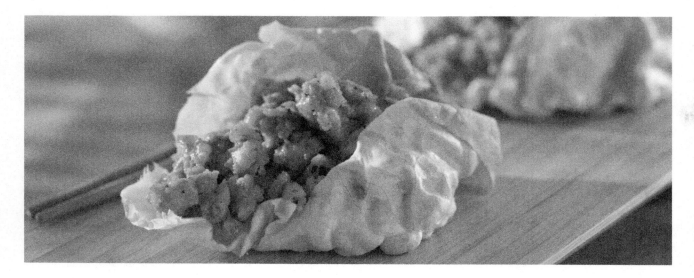

INGREDIENTS

- 1 tbsp. coconut oil
- 1 lb. ground chicken
- 2 tbsp. low-sodium soy sauce
- ¼ cup hoisin sauce
- 2 tbsp. unseasoned rice wine vinegar
- 1 tbsp. sriracha
- 2 tsp. freshly grated ginger
- 2 garlic cloves, minced
- 1 (8-ounce) can water chestnuts, drained and diced
- Butter lettuce leaves for serving

DIRECTIONS

1. In a large skillet over medium heat, heat the coconut oil.

2. Add the chicken, and cook thoroughly, using a spatula to break into crumbs.

3. Add the soy sauce, hoisin sauce, vinegar, and sriracha. Stir to combine and cook for 5 minutes or until most of the liquid has been absorbed.

4. Add the ginger, garlic, and water chestnuts, and cook for 1 minute.

5. Scoop 2 to 3 tablespoons of chicken mixture into each lettuce leaf to serve.

NUTRITION (per serving): Calories: 162 kcal | Fats: 2g | Carbs: 8g | Protein: 25g.

106. GRILLED CHICKEN WINGS

 15 min

 20 min

 Poultry Mains

 2 Servings

INGREDIENTS

- 1½ lb. frozen chicken wings
- Freshly ground black pepper
- 1 tsp. garlic powder
- 1 cup buffalo wing sauce, such as Frank's RedHot
- 1 tsp. extra-virgin olive oil.

DIRECTIONS

1. Preheat the grill to 350°F.
2. Season the wings with black pepper and garlic powder.
3. Grill the wings for 15 minutes per side. They will be browned and crispy when finished.
4. Toss the grilled wings in the buffalo wing sauce and olive oil.
5. Serve immediately.

NUTRITION (per serving): Calories: 82 kcal | Fats: 6g | Carbs: 1g | Protein: 7g.

107. MOIST CHICKEN DELUXE

 15 min

 80 min

 Poultry Mains

 12 Servings

INGREDIENTS

- 3 lb. chicken breasts, boneless and skinless
- 1¼ cups whole wheat Italian breadcrumbs
- ½ cup light mayonnaise dressing.

DIRECTIONS

1. Heat the oven over 425°.
2. Using a culinary brush, apply mayonnaise to the chicken breasts.
3. Put Italian bread crumbs into a separate plate and roll the chicken breasts over it until fully coated.
4. Next, use an aluminum foil pan and place the chicken breasts. Bake for about 40 to 45 minutes, or until the meat temperature reaches 165°F

NUTRITION (per serving): Calories: 320 kcal | Fats: 6g | Carbs: 41,3g | Protein: 28g.

108. TURKEY ROULADE WITH SPINACH

15 min

55 min

Poultry Mains

4-6 Servings

INGREDIENTS

- 1 tbsp. olive oil
- 1 turkey breast, boneless and skinless, butterflied
- 6 oz. baby spinach, rinsed
- 1 garlic clove, minced
- ¼ large onion, chopped
- ½ cup low-fat mozzarella cheese, grated
- 2 tbsp. breadcrumbs or oatmeal
- ¼ tsp. oregano, dried
- ¼ tsp. rosemary, dried
- ½ tsp. salt
- ½ tsp. ground black pepper
- 1 egg white
- 4 tbsp. chicken broth
- 10-12 cups of boiling water to blanch (flash cook) the spinach.

DIRECTIONS

1. Preheat the oven to 325°F.
2. Blanch the spinach in a large pot filled with boiling water. Cook for 30-60 seconds or just until wilted. Remove from the heat and place it in a colander. Drain and press the cooked spinach to remove excessive water. Set aside.
3. Coat a medium saucepan with olive oil. Sauté onion and garlic over medium heat. Cook for 2 minutes.
4. Add spinach, rosemary, oregano, salt and pepper. Continue cooking for another minute. Sir occasionally. Remove from heat. Let the spinach mixture rest for 5 minutes or until warm to touch.
5. In a large bowl, combine the spinach mixture with breadcrumbs, cheese, and egg white together. Mix well.
6. Take the butterflied boneless turkey breast, cover with plastic wrap, and start pounding to a roughly ¼ to ½ inch thickness by using a rolling pin or meat mallet. Discard the plastic wrap.
7. Place the spinach and cheese mixture in the center of turkey breast. Then roll up the breast to resemble a cigar. Season the surface of the turkey roll with salt and pepper.
8. Secure the turkey roll with baking twine.
9. Place the turkey roll on a baking dish/sheet. Carefully pour the chicken broth into a baking dish. Cover loosely with aluminum foil. Bake for 40 minutes or until the inner temperature reach 165°F.
10. Remove the aluminum foil and continue baking for additional 7 minutes or until the outer layer of the turkey turns golden brown.

NUTRITION (per serving): Calories: 181 kcal | Fats: 5.9g | Carbs: 2.8g | Protein: 17.4g.

109. CHICKEN MEATLOAF

15 min

40 min

Poultry Mains

1 Loaf

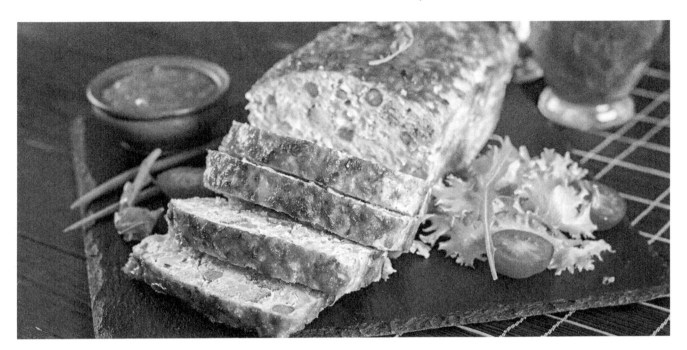

INGREDIENTS

- 1 lb. ground chicken breasts
- ¼ cup onion, minced
- ½ cup breadcrumbs or panko
- 1 egg
- ¼ cup celery, minced
- ¼ cup carrot, minced
- 2 cloves garlic, minced
- 3 tbsp. parsley, chopped
- ½ tsp. salt
- ½ tsp. black pepper
- Few tbsp. of chicken broth.

DIRECTIONS

1. Preheat the oven to 350°F.

2. Spray the baking dish with oil to prevent sticking.

3. Mix all the ingredients in a large bowl.

4. Add a few tablespoons of chicken broth to make the meatloaf mixture moist but not watery.

5. Transfer the meatloaf mixture to a baking dish. Cook for 40 minutes or until the loaf is fully cooked / inner temperature reach 165°F.

NUTRITION (per serving): Calories: 124.9 kcal | Fats: 5g | Carbs: 8.6g | Protein: 11.6g.

110. GREEK CHICKEN BITES

| 5 min | 20 min | Poultry Mains | 4 Servings |

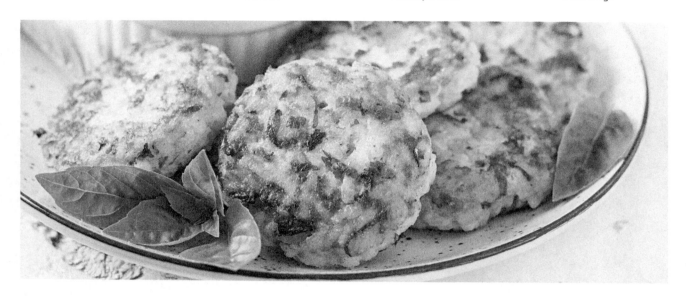

INGREDIENTS

- 1 lb. chicken thighs, boneless and skinless
- ½ small onion, diced
- 3 garlic cloves, peeled
- 1 egg white
- 1 tbsp. lemon juice
- 1½ tsp. Cavender's Greek Seasoning (otherwise use, 1 tsp. salt and ½ tsp. black pepper)
- A few dashes cayenne pepper
- 1 cup raw baby spinach, roughly chopped
- 1 tbsp. olive oil.

DIRECTIONS

1. Pulse the chicken, onion, garlic, egg white, lemon juice, seasoning and cayenne in a food processor until well combined but there is still some texture - do not make a smooth puree.

2. Transfer the ground mixture to a bowl and fold in the chopped spinach.

3. Portion into bite sized balls using a small metal scoop if you have one, otherwise use a teaspoon - dampen hands, roll into balls then flatten slightly.

4. Heat oil in a nonstick skillet and sauce the bites until golden, flip and cook an additional minute.

5. Remove to plate and serve with salad.

NUTRITION (per serving): Calories: 168 kcal | Fats: 6g | Carbs: 1g | Protein: 26g.

111. DELICIOUS TURKEY BURGER

15 min

15 min

Poultry Mains

6 Servings

INGREDIENTS

- 3 lb. ground turkey
- ¼ cup seasoned breadcrumbs
- ¼ cup onion, finely diced
- 2 egg whites, lightly beaten
- ¼ cup fresh parsley, chopped
- 1 garlic clove, minced
- Salt and ground black pepper.

DIRECTIONS

1. In a large bowl, mix ground turkey, seasoned breadcrumbs, onion, egg whites, parsley, garlic, salt, and pepper.

2. Form into 6 patties.

3. Cook the patties in a medium skillet over medium heat, turning once, to an internal temperature of 180°F.

NUTRITION (per serving): Calories: 184 kcal | Fats: 9.5g | Carbs: 2.3g | Protein: 20.9g.

112. CHICKEN & ZUCCHINI CASSEROLE

15 min

15 min

Poultry Mains

6 Servings

INGREDIENTS

- 3 medium zucchini, quartered
- 1½ lb. chicken breasts
- 1 (28-oz.) can diced tomatoes
- ½ cup pepperoncini peppers
- ¼ cup black olives, halved
- 1 tsp. Italian seasoning
- Sea salt and black pepper
- 1 cup shredded Italian cheese: Mozzarella, Provolone, Fontina blend.

DIRECTIONS

1. Preheat oven to 375°F.

2. Cut zucchini, pepperoncini peppers and chicken breasts into 1-inch cubes. Drain tomatoes.

3. In a large baking dish toss the chicken, zucchini, peppers, olives, Italian seasoning, tomatoes, salt and pepper.

4. Cover with foil and bake for 35 to 45 minutes, until chicken is just cooked through. Remove foil add cheese and bake until cheese is melted, 8 to 10 minutes.

NUTRITION (per serving): Calories: 268 kcal | Fats: 20g | Carbs: 11 g | Protein: 12g.

113. CHICKEN TIKKA MASALA

20 min   55 min   Poultry Mains   6 Servings

Creamy and tangy chicken stew cooked on a stove top.
This recipe comes with homemade garam marsala recipe, but you can get a store-bought version at spices section or Indian/specialty store.

INGREDIENTS

- 1 lb. chicken breasts, boneless and skinless, cut into chunks
- 1 medium onion, chopped
- 3 tbsp. minced ginger
- 6 cloves garlic, minced
- Salt and ground black pepper
- 2 tsp. olive oil
- 2 tsp. smoked paprika
- 3 tbsp. tomato paste
- 1 tbsp. garam masala
- ½ cup of nonfat milk (or 2 tbsp. thick unsweetened coconut milk)
- 1 cup nonfat yogurt
- 1 cup water

FOR GARAM MARSALA
- 2 tsp. ground cumin
- 1 tsp. ground coriander
- 1 tsp. ground cardamom
- 1 tsp. ground black pepper
- ½ tsp. ground cinnamon
- ¼ tsp. ground cloves
- ¼ tsp. ground nutmeg.

DIRECTIONS

1. In a large saucepan, over medium heat, sauté onion and chicken chunks with olive oil for 5 minutes.

2. Sprinkle minced garlic, ginger, and tomato paste into the chicken mixture. Mix well. Cook for 1 minute.

3. Stir in salt, pepper, paprika, garam masala, yogurt, milk, and water. Bring to boil. Stir occasionally.

4. Lower the heat, cover with a lid, and simmer for 20-25 minutes or until the chicken is cooked and the sauce is thickened.

5. Garnish with chopped cilantro, if desired.

TO MAKE GARAM MARSALA

6. Combine all ingredients in an airtight container. Mix well and store in a cool, dry place.

NUTRITION (per serving): Calories: 295.4 kcal | Fats: 15.4g | Carbs: 13.7g | Protein: 26.2g.

Chapter 12

BEEF & PORK MAINS RECIPES

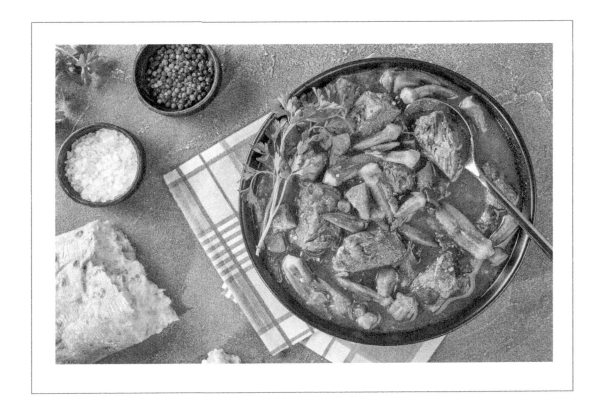

114. ZOODLES WITH MEAT SAUCE

| 10 min | 40 min | Beef & Pork Mains | 4 Servings |

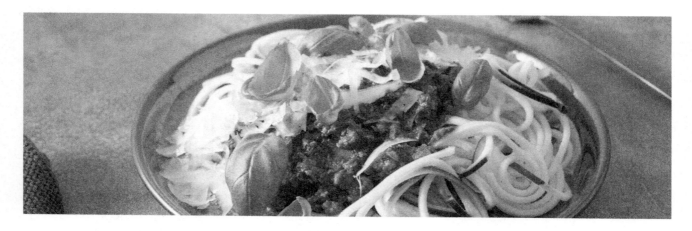

INGREDIENTS

- 1 lb. ground beef (93%)
- 2 tbsp. extra-virgin olive oil
- 1 large yellow onion, chopped
- 3 garlic cloves, minced
- 1 tbsp. tomato paste
- 1 (24-ounce) jar pasta sauce
- 1 tbsp. Italian seasoning
- 4 medium zucchini
- ½ cup Parmesan cheese, shredded.

DIRECTIONS

1. In a large saucepan over medium heat, cook the ground beef, breaking it up with the spoon, until browned, 7 to 10 minutes. Drain, and transfer to a plate.

2. In the same pan over medium heat, heat 1 tablespoon of oil. Add the onions and garlic, and sauté until the onions are translucent and the garlic is fragrant, about 5 minutes. Add the tomato paste, and sauté for 1 minute.

3. Add the pasta sauce and stir well to combine. Mix in the Italian seasoning. Simmer for 20 minutes.

4. Meanwhile, cut the zucchini noodles to their desired length.

5. In a large skillet over medium heat, heat the remaining tablespoon of oil. Add the zucchini, and sauté until soft, 2 to 3 minutes, or to desired texture. Be sure not to overcook the zucchini, as it will end up mushy.

6. Plate the zucchini, top with the sauce and Parmesan, and serve.

NUTRITION (per serving): Calories: 410 kcal | Fats: 20g | Carbs: 26g | Protein: 32g.

115. SLOW COOKER PULLED PORK

5 min

6 h

Beef & Pork Mains

8 Servings

INGREDIENTS

- 1 onion, cut into thick rings
- 1 (4-pound) pork shoulder, trimmed
- 1 tbsp. salt
- 1 tsp. black pepper
- 1 tsp. garlic powder
- 1 tsp. onion powder
- 1 tbsp. paprika
- 2 tbsp. extra-virgin olive oil.

DIRECTIONS

1. Cover the bottom of a 4-to 6-quart slow cooker with the onion slices and place the pork on top.
2. In a small bowl combine the salt, pepper, garlic powder, onion powder, paprika, and olive oil. Rub the mixture over the pork.
3. Cook on high for 4 to 6 hours or on low for 7 to 8 hours or until tender.
4. Discard the excess fat and onions. Shred the pork with two forks, and serve with your favorite sauce.

NUTRITION (per serving): Calories: 562 kcal | Fats: 34g | Carbs: 2g | Protein: 58g.

116. CHIPOTLE SHREDDED PORK

10 min

6 h

Beef & Pork Mains

8 Servings

INGREDIENTS

- 1 (7.5-ounce) can chipotle peppers in adobo sauce
- 1½ tbsp. apple cider vinegar
- 1 tbsp. ground cumin
- 1 tbsp. dried oregano
- 1 lime juice
- 2 lb. pork shoulder, trimmed of excess fat

DIRECTIONS

1. In a blender or food processor, puree the chipotle peppers and adobo sauce, apple cider vinegar, cumin, oregano, and lime juice.
2. Place the pork shoulder in the slow cooker and pour the sauce over it. Cover the slow cooker and cook on low for 6 hours.
3. The finished pork should shred easily. Use two forks to shred the pork in the slow cooker. If there is any additional sauce, allow the pork to cook on low for 20 minutes more to absorb the remaining liquid.

NUTRITION (per serving): Calories: 260 kcal | Fats: 11g | Carbs: 5g | Protein: 20g.

117. BEEF STEW
WITH RUTABAGA & CARROTS

15 min

40 min

Beef & Pork Mains

3 Servings

This rich, hearty beef stew has a garden full of flavor
with vegetables like rutabaga and carrots.
You can throw in extra vegetables to stretch it.

INGREDIENTS

- 4 tsp. extra-virgin olive oil
- 1 lb. beef sirloin steak, cut into 1-inch cubes
- 2 tsp. garlic, minced
- 1 medium onion, chopped
- 1 lb. rutabaga, peeled and cut into ½-inch cubes
- 3 medium carrots, peeled and cut into ½-inch cubes
- 1 small tomato, diced
- 1 tsp. smoked paprika
- ½ tsp. ground coriander
- ¼ tsp. red pepper flakes
- 2 tbsp. whole-wheat flour
- ½ cup red wine
- 3 cups low-sodium beef broth
- Fresh minced parsley for garnish.

DIRECTIONS

1. In a large soup pot or Dutch oven, heat 2 teaspoons of olive oil over medium heat.

2. Add the beef and brown it on all sides, stirring frequently, until no longer pink, about 5 minutes. Transfer to a bowl and set aside.

3. In the same pot, heat the remaining 2 teaspoons of olive oil over medium heat. Add the garlic and onion, and cook, stirring frequently, until the onion is tender, 1 to 2 minutes.

4. Stir in the rutabaga, carrots, tomato, paprika, coriander, and red pepper flakes.

5. Add the flour and cook, stirring constantly, for 1 minute. Add the red wine and stir for an additional minute.

6. Add the broth and return the beef to the pot. Bring to a boil and then reduce the heat to low to simmer. The sauce should start to thicken.

7. Cover the pot and cook for 30 minutes, or until all the vegetables are tender.

8. Serve garnished with the parsley.

NUTRITION (per serving): Calories: 292 kcal | Fats: 13g | Carbs: 8g | Protein: 34g.

118. BELL PEPPER NACHOS

 10 min

 20 min

 Beef & Pork Mains

 4 Servings

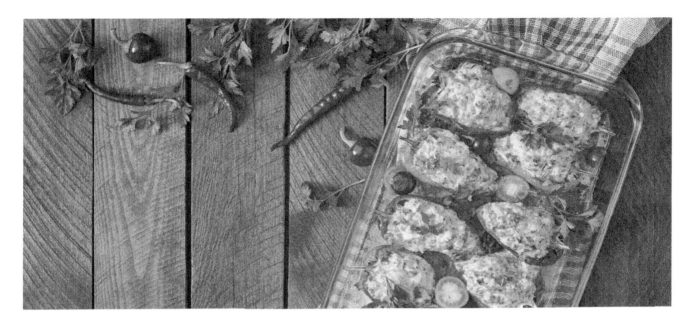

INGREDIENTS

- 1 lb. lean ground beef (93%)
- ⅓ cup salsa
- 2 tbsp. Taco Seasoning
- Nonstick cooking spray
- 20 to 25 mini bell peppers, halved lengthwise, trimmed, and seeded
- 1 cup Mexican cheese, shredded.

DIRECTIONS

1. Preheat the oven to 400°F.

2. In a large skillet over medium heat, brown the meat until no longer pink, breaking it up as it cooks, 7 to 10 minutes. Drain the meat and stir in the salsa and taco seasoning. Simmer for 3 to 5 minutes, until the liquid has cooked down.

3. Spray a large baking sheet with cooking spray and arrange the peppers on the sheet cut side up.

4. Fill the peppers with the beef, and sprinkle with the cheese.

5. Bake until the cheese is melted, about 5 minutes, and serve immediately

NUTRITION (per serving): Calories: 348 kcal | Fats: 17g | Carbs: 15g | Protein: 31g.

119. HAWAIIAN PORK KABOBS WITH PINEAPPLE

 15 min 20 min Beef & Pork Mains 4 Servings

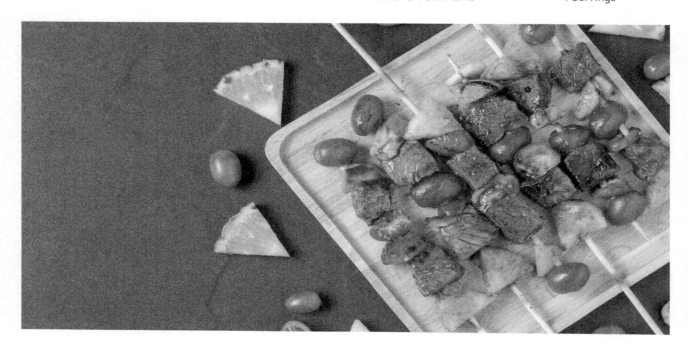

INGREDIENTS

- ¼ cup low-sodium soy sauce
- 3 tbsp. extra-virgin olive oil
- 2 garlic cloves, minced
- Salt and black pepper
- 1 lb. pork loin, diced into 1½-inch cubes
- 1½ cups pineapple chunks
- 1 white onion, peeled and chopped into 1-inch pieces
- 1 red bell pepper, trimmed,

DIRECTIONS

1. Prepare 8 to 10 wooden skewers by soaking them in water for 15 minutes to prevent burning. If you are using metal skewers, you can skip this step.

2. In a large bowl, whisk the soy sauce, 2 tablespoons of olive oil, garlic, and salt and pepper to taste. Add the pork chunks to the bowl and toss to coat. Cover and chill for at least 15 minutes.

3. Carefully thread the skewers with the pork, pineapple, onions, and peppers, repeating until all the ingredients are used.

4. Lightly brush the pork and vegetables with the remaining tablespoon of olive oil.

seeded, and cut into 1-inch pieces

- 1 yellow pepper, trimmed, seeded, and cut into 1-inch pieces.

5. Heat the grill to high, then reduce to 400°F.

6. Place the kabobs on the grill. Cook for 3 to 4 minutes, rotate, and repeat until all sides are browned, and the pork is cooked through to 145°F. Serve immediately.

NUTRITION (per serving): Calories: 292 kcal | Fats: 15g | Carbs: 17g | Protein: 24g.

120. ONE-PAN PORK CHOPS WITH APPLES & RED ONION

 10 min

 30 min

 Beef & Pork Mains

 4 Servings

INGREDIENTS

- 2 tsp. extra-virgin olive oil
- 4 boneless center-cut thin pork chops
- 2 small apples, thinly sliced
- 1 small red onion, thinly sliced
- 1 cup low-sodium chicken broth
- 1 tsp. Dijon mustard
- 1 tsp. dried sage
- 1 tsp. dried thyme.

DIRECTIONS

1. Place a large nonstick frying pan over high heat and add 1 teaspoon of olive oil. When the oil is hot, add the pork chops and reduce the heat to medium. Sear the chops for 3 minutes on one side, flip, and sear the other side for 3 minutes, 6 minutes total. Transfer the chops to a plate and set aside.

2. In the same pan, add the remaining 1 teaspoon of olive oil. Add the apples and onion. Cook for 5 minutes or until tender, stirring frequently to prevent burning.

3. While the apples and onion cook, mix together the broth and Dijon mustard in a small bowl.

4. Add the sage and thyme to the pan and stir to coat the onion and apples. Stir in the broth mixture and return the pork chops to the pan. Cover the pan and simmer for 10 to 15 minutes.

5. Let pork chops rest for 2 minutes before cutting.

NUTRITION (per serving): Calories: 234 kcal | Fats: 11g | Carbs: 13g | Protein: 20g.

121. PORK TENDERLOIN WITH ROASTED GREEN BEANS

 10 min

 30 min

 Beef & Pork Mains

 3 Servings

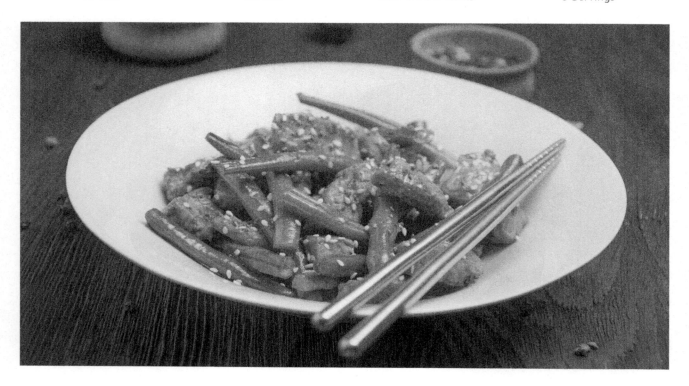

INGREDIENTS

- 2 tbsp. whole grain mustard
- 2 tbsp. honey
- 2 tbsp. soy sauce
- 2 garlic cloves, minced
- 1 tbsp. sriracha
- Salt and black pepper
- 1 lb. fresh green beans, trimmed

DIRECTIONS

1. Preheat the oven to 450°F. Line a baking sheet with aluminum foil.

2. In a small bowl, mix the mustard, honey, soy sauce, garlic, and sriracha. Season with salt and pepper to taste.

3. Place the green beans on the prepared baking sheet and toss with the olive oil.

4. Place the pork on top of the green beans. Rub half of the sauce on the pork evenly.

5. Bake for 15 minutes, then remove from oven. Brush the

- 1 tbsp. extra-virgin olive oil
- 1 lb. trimmed pork tenderloin
- 2 tbsp. sesame seeds for garnish.

remaining sauce over the pork. Return the pork to the oven and cook for another 10 to 15 minutes, or until the internal temperature of the pork is between 145-150°F and the meat is pale and mostly white with mostly clear juices.

6. Remove from the oven. Garnish with sesame seeds. Tent the pork with foil.

7. Let rest for 10 to 15 minutes before serving.

NUTRITION (per serving): Calories: 313 kcal | Fats: 9g | Carbs: 26g | Protein: 36g.

122. BEEF & BROCCOLI STIR-FRY

10 min

1 h 20 min

Beef & Pork Mains

4 Servings

INGREDIENTS

- 1 lb. flat iron steak
- 1 tbsp. cornstarch
- ½ cup soy sauce
- ¼ cup oyster sauce
- ½ cup beef broth
- 1 tbsp. minced fresh ginger
- 2 garlic cloves, minced
- 5 cups broccoli florets
- 1 tbsp. coconut oil
- Cauliflower rice (optional).

DIRECTIONS

1. Thinly slice the flat iron steak against the grain.

2. In a large, resealable bag, toss the meat with the cornstarch. Add the soy sauce, oyster sauce, beef broth, ginger, and garlic. Chill for 1 hour.

3. In a large pot, blanch the broccoli for 2 minutes in boiling water, then transfer to an ice bath.

4. In a large wok or skillet over medium-high heat, heat the oil. Add the beef (reserve remaining marinade), and stir-fry until brown, 1 to 3 minutes. Transfer to a plate.

5. Add the blanched broccoli to the wok or skillet, and stir-fry until crisp but tender, about 3 minutes. Add the remaining marinade and cook for 2 minutes more.

6. Return the beef to the pan with the broccoli, and warm through.

7. Serve with cauliflower rice (if desired).

NUTRITION (per serving): Calories: 348 kcal per serving | Fats: 17g | Carbs: 31g | Protein: 15g.

123. ITALIAN MEATLOAF

 20 min

 1 h

 Beef & Pork Mains

 10 Servings

INGREDIENTS

FOR THE MEATLOAF

- 2 tbsp. olive oil
- 1 medium onion, diced
- 3 garlic cloves, minced
- 1 large red pepper, diced
- 1 lb. ground sirloin
- ¼ cup oatmeal
- 1/3 cup breadcrumbs (or panko bread)
- ¾ cup Parmagiano Reggiano cheese, grated
- 2 eggs
- 1 tbsp. Worcestershire sauce
- 1 tbsp. balsamic vinegar
- 2 tbsp. basil leaves, chopped
- 1 tbsp. fresh parsley, chopped

FOR THE GLAZE/SAUCE

- ½ cup marinara sauce

-OR MADE FROM SCRATCH VERSION-

- ½ cup ketchup
- 1 tsp. ground cumin
- ¼ tsp. Worcestershire sauce
- ¼ tsp. hot sauce/ tabasco
- 1 tbsp. honey.

DIRECTIONS

TO MAKE MEATLOAF

1. Preheat oven to 350 degrees.

2. In a medium sized pan, sauté onion, pepper and garlic with olive oil over medium heat. Cook until the vegetables are soft.

3. Remove from heat. Let it cool for few minutes.

4. Add the remaining ingredients and combine.

5. Shape the mixture into a loaf on a pre-oiled or parchment paper-lined baking sheet.

6. Bake for 45 - 55 minutes or until the inner temperature reaches 155 degrees.

7. Spread the marinara sauce or homemade glaze sauce on top of the meatloaf. Place back in the oven to for 10 minutes.

8. Allow the fully cooked meatloaf to rest for about 5 minutes.

TO MAKE HOMEMADE GLAZE

9. Combine cumin, ketchup, honey, hot sauce, and Worcestershire sauce together. Mix well to even consistency.

NUTRITION (per serving): Calories: 300 kcal | Fats: 15.9g | Carbs: 10.6g | Protein: 18.9g.

124. LAMB KEBABS WITH CUCUMBER DIPPING SAUCE

10 min

25 min

Beef & Pork Mains

6 Servings

INGREDIENTS

- 1 medium onion, diced
- 3 garlic cloves, minced
- Olive oil
- 1 tsp. ground cumin
- 2 tsp. fresh oregano leaves (or 1 teaspoon dried oregano)
- ¼ tsp. crushed red pepper or cayenne pepper
- 1 lb. ground lamb
- ½ cup chopped flat leaf parsley
- 1 lemon zest and juice
- Sea salt
- Freshly ground black pepper
- ½ cup plain Greek yogurt, not fat free, use real yogurt
- ¼ cup diced cucumber
- ½ small jalapeño, stem and seeds removed.

DIRECTIONS

1. Sauté the onion and 1 teaspoon of the minced garlic in 1 tablespoon olive oil over medium high heat in a small skillet until tender.

2. Add 1 teaspoon cumin, oregano, red pepper flakes and cook, stirring, for another minute - set aside to cool slightly.

3. Combine the lamb in a large mixing bowl with the onion mixture, chopped parsley and lemon zest along with 1 tablespoon olive oil, 1 teaspoon salt and 1/2 teaspoon black pepper.

4. Divide the mixture into pieces the size of golf balls and flatten two of them into a thick patty around a bamboo skewer - arrange on a platter, cover and chill for about 10 minutes to firm. This makes 6 skewers.

5. Meanwhile, make the dressing by combining the yogurt, cucumber, remaining 1/2 teaspoon minced garlic, 1 tablespoon of the lemon juice, 1/2 teaspoon cumin, jalapeño, 1/2 teaspoon salt, 1/4 teaspoon black pepper in the blender until smooth. pour into small bowl and set aside. You can also combine in a bowl for a salsa style creamy sauce.

6. Preheat grill or grill pan and cook the lamb kebabs for 5 to 6 minutes, turning halfway through so that both sides are well browned. I grill slices of onion and sweet pepper alongside the lamb.

7. Serve warm with the dressing on the side. These are delicious.

NUTRITION (per serving): Calories: 148 kcal | Fats: 8.7g | Carbs: 4.3g | Protein: 13g.

125. MAGICALLY SAVORY PORK

10 min

6 h

Beef & Pork Mains

8 Servings

INGREDIENTS

- 1 lb. lean pork tenderloins, cut into thin strips
- 2 tbsp. corn starch
- ½ tsp. salt
- Nonstick cooking spray
- ⅓ cup wine vinegar
- ½ cup water
- 1 (15-oz.) can pineapple chunks (unsweetened)
- ¼ cup brown sugar
- 1 tbsp. soy sauce (low sodium)
- 2 medium green peppers, sized and finely slice
- 3 cups brown rice, cooked
- 1 small-sized onions, chopped.

DIRECTIONS

1. Prepare a nonstick cooking pan and apply with cooking spray. Heat the pan over medium-high temperature.

2. Next, is to place the pork onto the pan and cook until golden brown consistency is achieved.

3. After the pork becomes golden brown, remove and put it on a separate plate. Set it aside for a moment.

4. Drain excess fats from the cooking pan.

5. Get the pineapple chunks can and separate the liquid from the chunks. Set aside pineapple juice for a moment.

6. Prepare a small bowl and combine soy sauce, brown sugar, water, pineapple juice, salt, vinegar, and cornstarch. Stir for about 1 to 3 minutes.

7. Add it to the cooking pan and cook for about 2 minutes or it until the sauce becomes dense.

8. And then, add the pork loins and cook over a low temperature for about 30 minutes, or until meat is tender. Stir the dish occasionally.

9. Finish the process by adding pineapple chunks, onions, and peppers. Cook it for another 5 minutes.

10. Serve the dish with rice.

NUTRITION (per serving): Calories: 227 kcal | Fats: 8,9g | Carbs: 8g | Protein: 27,7g.

Chapter 13

VEGETABLES & SIDES RECIPES

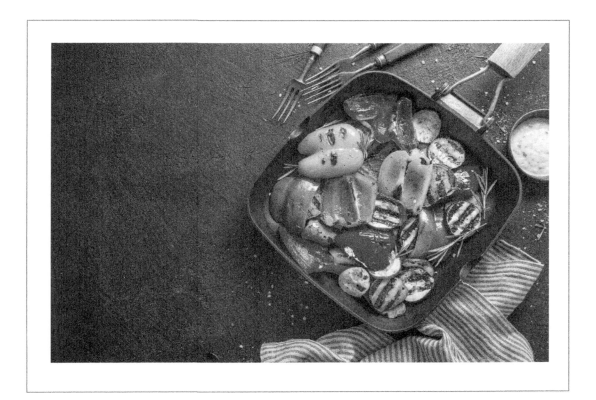

126. ROASTED GARDEN VEGETABLES

5 min   35 min   Vegetables & Sides   6 Servings

INGREDIENTS

- 1 medium bell pepper, cut into strips
- 1 small onion, halved, sliced
- 1 small zucchini, sliced into rounds
- 1-pint grape tomatoes
- 2 tbsp. extra-virgin olive oil
- Salt and black pepper.

DIRECTIONS

1. Preheat the oven to 400°F. Using 1 or 2 large baking sheets, arrange the vegetables, so they are lying flat, lightly touching each other.
2. Evenly pour the olive oil over the vegetables and gently toss to coat, using either a spoon or your hands. Add salt and pepper to taste.
3. Roast for 20 to 30 minutes, or until soft and lightly charred, stirring halfway through, and serve.

NUTRITION (per serving): Calories: 75 kcal | Fats: 5g | Carbs: 0g | Protein: 8g.

127. ROASTED ROOT VEGETABLES

15 min   45 min   Vegetables & Sides   6 Servings

INGREDIENTS

- 2 medium red beets, peeled
- 2 large parsnips, peeled
- 2 large carrots, peeled
- 1 medium butternut squash (about 2 pounds), peeled and seeded
- 1 medium red onion
- 2 tbsp. extra-virgin olive oil
- 4 tsp. garlic, minced
- 2 tsp. dried thyme.

DIRECTIONS

1. Roughly chop the beets, parsnips, carrots, and butternut squash into 1-inch pieces. Cut the onion into half and then each half into 4 large chunks.
2. Preheat the oven to 425°F. Spray a large, rimmed baking sheet with the cooking spray. Arrange the vegetables in a single, even layer on the baking sheet, and sprinkle them with olive oil, garlic, and thyme. Use a spoon to mix the vegetables to coat them with the oil and seasonings.
3. Roast for 45 minutes, stirring the vegetables every 15 minutes, until all the vegetables are tender. Serve immediately.

NUTRITION (per serving): Calories: 115 kcal | Fats: 9g | Carbs: 4g | Protein: 6g.

128. OVEN-ROASTED BABY CARROTS

| 10 min | 1 h | Vegetables & Sides | 6 Servings |

INGREDIENTS

- 1 lb. baby carrots
- 2 tbsp. olive oil
- ½ tsp. dried oregano
- 2 tbsp. freshly chopped parsley
- Salt and ground pepper
- 1 tsp. honey.

DIRECTIONS

1. Preheat the oven to 375°F. In a large bowl, toss carrots with oregano, salt, pepper, parsley, olive oil and honey.
2. Spread carrots evenly on a large parchment-lined baking sheet.
3. Cover loosely with foil. Bake carrots for 45 minutes or until the carrots are tender. Remove the foil and continue baking for 10 minutes.
4. Season with salt and pepper to taste.

NUTRITION (per serving): Calories: 109 kcal | Fats: 5.8g | Carbs: 14g | Protein: 1.4g.

129. SAUTÉED MUSHROOMS

| 10 min | 5 min | Vegetables & Sides | 6 Servings |

INGREDIENTS

- 1 lb. of Cremini or white mushrooms, rinsed well
- ¼ medium onion, chopped
- 1 bell pepper, seeded, sliced
- 3 garlic cloves, minced
- 1 tsp. ginger, minced
- ¼ cup low-sodium soy sauce
- 1 tbsp. olive oil
- 2 tbsp. fresh parsley, chopped
- 1 tbsp. lemon juice
- Pinch of salt and pepper.

DIRECTIONS

1. In a large wok or nonstick skillet, stir-fry onion, bell pepper, garlic, ginger, and mushrooms with olive oil over high heat for 1-2 minutes.
2. Add soy sauce and lemon juice. Stir well. Cook for additional 30-60 seconds.
3. Sprinkle parsley leaves and season with salt and pepper to taste.

NUTRITION (per serving): Calories: 76 kcal | Fats: 6.6g | Carbs: 3.8g | Protein: 1.2g.

130. CAULIFLOWER COUSCOUS

 5 min

 15 min

 Vegetables & Sides

 6 Servings

INGREDIENTS

- 1 cauliflower head, cut into large chunks
- 2 tbsp. olive oil
- 1 tbsp. grated lemon zest
- 1 tsp. fresh lemon juice
- 1 tsp. minced fresh parsley
- 1 tablespoon minced fresh mint
- Salt and paper, to taste.

DIRECTIONS

1. Rinse and trim cauliflower's leaves and stem. Cut cauliflower into large chunks. Pulse in a food processor, until small grains are formed.

2. In a large nonstick skillet, sauté cauliflower with 1 tablespoon of olive oil over medium heat for 1 minute. Add a pinch of salt and mix well. Lower the heat, cover the skillet with a lid, and continue cooking for 5-10 minutes, until tender but still grainy.

3. Stir in the oil, lemon zest, lemon juice, and herbs. Season with salt and pepper to taste.

NUTRITION (per serving): Calories: 82 kcal | Fats: 7g | Carbs: 5g | Protein: 1g.

131. CURRIED CAULIFLOWER

 15 min

 35 min

 Vegetables & Sides

 6 Servings

INGREDIENTS

- 1 head cauliflower, cut into medium florets
- 1 tbsp. olive oil
- 1 tsp. ground cumin
- ½ tsp. ground cardamom
- 1 tbsp. curry powder
- Salt and black pepper
- Cooking spray.

DIRECTIONS

1. Preheat the oven to 375°F.

2. In a large bowl, combine all ingredients together. Mix well.

3. Spray and coat a baking dish/sheet with a cooking spray.

4. Place the seasoned cauliflower florets, spread into a single layer on the baking sheet/dish, and bake for 30-35 minutes or until tender.

NUTRITION (per serving): Calories: 126 kcal | Fats: 5g | Carbs: 9g | Protein: 9g.

132. CREAMY CAULIFLOWER

15 min

10 min

Vegetables & Sides

4 Servings

INGREDIENTS

- 1 medium cauliflower head, chopped
- 2 garlic cloves, peeled, whole
- Sea salt
- Freshly ground black pepper
- ¼ cup chicken broth
- 1 tbsp. olive oil
- ¼ cup plain Greek yogurt
- 2 green onions (or chives), chopped.

DIRECTIONS

1. Add the cauliflower, garlic and a pinch of salt to a boiling pot of water, cover and cook until very tender, 8 to 10 minutes.

2. Drain well then dry by turning out onto paper towels and pressing down with more paper towels - this is a key step.

3. Add the hot cauliflower and garlic cloves to a food processor with the broth, olive oil, and yogurt - process until very smooth.

4. Stir in a pinch of salt and pepper to taste and top with the chopped green onions or chives.

NUTRITION (per serving): Calories: 128 kcal | Fats: 7.8g | Carbs: 7g | Protein: 7,7g.

133. CREAMY SPINACH

13 min

17 min

Vegetables & Sides

3 Servings

INGREDIENTS

- 2 garlic cloves, peeled and minced
- 8 oz. spinach leaves
- 4 tbsp. sour cream
- 1 tbsp. butter
- 2 tbsp. Parmesan cheese, grated.

DIRECTIONS

1. Preheat pan with the oil over medium heat, add the spinach, stir and cook until it softens.

2. Add the salt, pepper, butter, Parmesan cheese, and butter, stir, and cook for 4 minutes. Add the sour cream, stir, and cook for 5 minutes.

3. Divide between plates and serve.

NUTRITION (per serving): Calories: 77 kcal | Fats: 10g | Carbs: 5.4g | Protein: 6.1g.

134. ASIAN PEANUT CABBAGE SLAW

 10 min
 10 min
 Vegetables & Sides
 4 Servings

INGREDIENTS

- 1 (14-ounce) package coleslaw
- 1 red bell pepper, thinly sliced
- 1 large carrot, grated
- ¼ cup diced scallions
- ¼ cup chopped fresh cilantro
- ¼ cup chopped peanuts
- ⅓ cup Spicy Peanut Dressing, plus more if desired.

DIRECTIONS

1. In a large bowl, combine coleslaw, bell pepper, carrot, scallions, cilantro, and peanuts. Toss with the dressing, add more as desired, and serve.

NUTRITION (per serving): Calories: 123 kcal | Fats: 6g | Carbs: 6g | Protein: 16g.

135. GRILLED ASPARAGUS

 15 min
 35 min
 Vegetables & Sides
 6 Servings

INGREDIENTS

- 1 lb. fresh asparagus
- Olive oil
- Sea salt and freshly ground black pepper
- 1 lemon.

DIRECTIONS

1. Snap off the bottom cut end of each asparagus and peel the bottom 2-inches with a vegetable peeler. Lightly coat the asparagus with olive oil, salt and pepper by rolling them around with your hands against each other on a large plate.

2. Heat a grill pan or skillet over medium high heat and cook the asparagus until marked with light brown and slightly softened, 3 to 4 minutes. Serve in a pile with a big lemon squeeze.

NUTRITION (per serving): Calories: 45.9 kcal | Fats: 2.5g | Carbs: 5.2g | Protein: 2.6g.

136. BALSAMIC WATERMELON & FETA SALAD

5 min

5 min

Vegetables & Sides

4 Servings

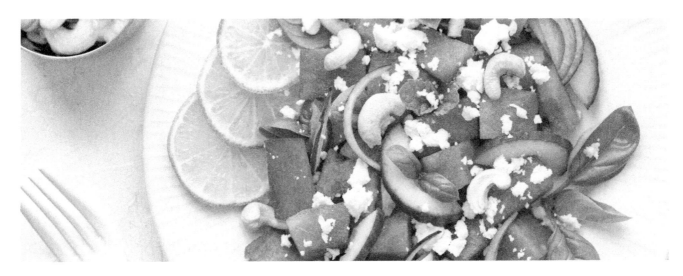

INGREDIENTS

- 4 cups watermelon in bite-sized chunks, seeds removed
- 2 oz. feta cheese, crumbled
- 2 tbsp. prepared balsamic vinaigrette dressing
- 1 cucumber, sliced
- 3 tbsp. fresh basil, chopped
- 3 tbsp. red onion, thinly sliced
- 3 tbsp. fresh mint, chopped
- 1 tsp. olive oil
- Salt and pepper, to taste.

DIRECTIONS

1. On a large platter or individual plates, arrange watermelon and feta.

2. Drizzle with vinaigrette and top with basil.

NUTRITION (per serving): Calories: 97 kcal | Fats: 3g | Carbs: 15g | Protein: 5g.

137. BROCCOLI APPLE SALAD

15 min

0 min

Vegetables & Sides

4 Servings

INGREDIENTS

- 2 cups broccoli florets
- ½ cup red onion, diced
- ¼ cup carrot, shredded
- 1 Gala apple, peeled, cored and diced
- ¼ cup pecans, chopped
- ⅓ cup Greek yogurt
- 2 tbsp. low-fat mayonnaise
- 2 tsp. lemon juice
- 2 tbsp. Splenda, granulated
- Salt and black pepper.

DIRECTIONS

1. Lightly steam or roast broccoli florets and let cool.

2. Toss the broccoli, onion, carrot, apple and pecans.

3. Blend the yogurt, mayonnaise, lemon juice, Splenda, salt and black pepper.

4. Pour the dressing over the salad and mix using two large spoons until lightly coated.

5. Serve chilled.

NUTRITION (per serving): Calories: 82.2 kcal | Fats: 2.4g | Carbs: 15.3g | Protein: 3.6g

138. ASIAN CUCUMBER SALAD

10 min

0 min

Vegetables & Sides

1 Servings

INGREDIENTS

- 1/4 cup Japanese rice vinegar
- ½ tsp. sesame oil
- Salt and red pepper, crushed
- 1 cucumber, shredded or sliced
- 1 cup cabbage, finely shredded
- 1 tbsp. sesame seeds, toasted.

DIRECTIONS

1. Blend rice vinegar, sesame oil, a pinch of salt, a pinch of crushed red pepper in a small bowl.

2. Toss with a cucumber and cabbage.

3. Top with toasted sesame seeds.

NUTRITION (per serving): Calories: 70.2 kcal | Fats: 1.1g | Carbs: 11.7g | Protein: 0.6g.

Chapter 14

SAUCES & SEASONINGS RECIPES

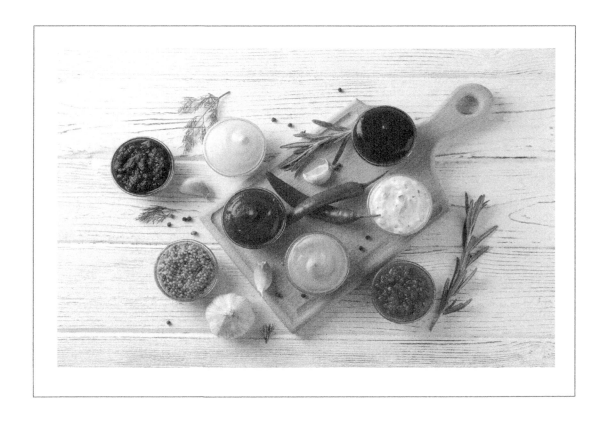

139. OIL-FREE VEGAN MAYONNAISE

1 h

5 min

Sauces & Seasonings

4 Servings

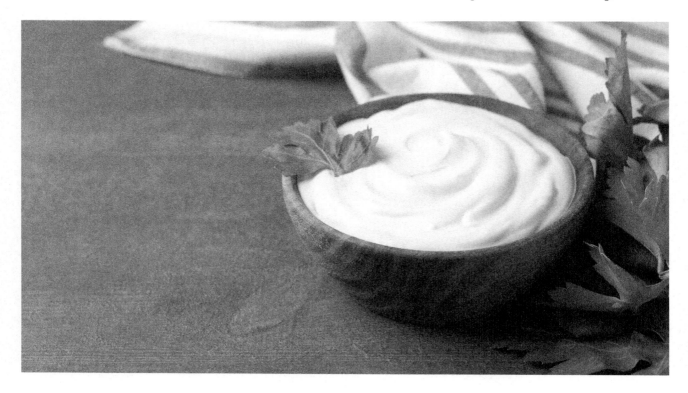

INGREDIENTS

- 1 cup raw unsalted cashews
- ½ cup hot water
- 1 tbsp + 1 tsp lemon juice
- ¼ tsp. Dijon mustard
- Sea salt, to taste.

DIRECTIONS

1. Soak cashews in hot water for at least 1 hour or in warm water overnight.

2. Drain and rinse the cashews and add them to a blender with the rest of the ingredients. Blend until smooth.

3. Adjust salt to taste.

4. Keep the mayo in a sealed container in the fridge for up to 5 days.

NUTRITION (per serving): Calories: 36 kcal | Fats: 2.9g | Carbs: 2.1g | Protein: 1g.

140. GREEK SALAD DRESSING

10 min

0 min

Sauces & Seasonings

2 Servings

INGREDIENTS

- ½ cup red wine vinegar
- ½ tsp. Dijon mustard
- ½ tsp. pepper
- 1 tsp. dried basil
- 1 tbsp. dried oregano
- 4 tsp. minced garlic
- 1 lemon juice
- ⅓ cup olive oil.

DIRECTIONS

1. Bring out a bowl and whisk together the mustard, pepper, basil, oregano, garlic, lemon juice, and olive oil.

2. Whisk in the red wine vinegar until it is emulsified. Pour into glasses and enjoy and store the leftovers in an airtight container.

NUTRITION (per serving): Calories: 89 kcal | Fats: 9g | Carbs: 1g | Protein: 0g.

141. MANGO SALSA

5 min

0 min

Sauces & Seasonings

2 Servings

INGREDIENTS

- ¼ red onion, diced
- 1 jalapeno pepper, stemmed and diced
- 2 limes juice
- ¼ cup cilantro, chopped
- 1 mango, diced and peeled.

DIRECTIONS

1. Bring out a bowl and add together the onion, jalapeno, lime juice, cilantro, and mango.

2. Use this right away or store overnight.

NUTRITION (per serving): Calories: 27 kcal | Fats: 0g | Carbs: 7g | Protein: 0g.

142. PESTO

10 min

0 min

Sauces & Seasonings

5 Servings

INGREDIENTS

- 1 tbsp. olive oil
- 2 garlic cloves
- 1 tbsp. dried basil
- 2 tbsp. grated Parmesan cheese
- ⅓ cup cottage cheese
- 1 packet spinach, chopped
- ½ cup water.

DIRECTIONS

1. Add all of these ingredients into the blender and then blend to make it all smooth.

2. Put on your favorite dish and enjoy it.

NUTRITION (per serving): Calories: 35 kcal | Fats: 1g | Carbs: 2g | Protein: 4g.

143. SEAFOOD SAUCE

10 min

0 min

Sauces & Seasonings

2 Servings

INGREDIENTS

- ¼ tsp. pepper
- 1 tsp. chili powder
- 1 tbsp. Worcestershire sauce
- 1 lemon juice
- 2 tbsp. horseradish, grated
- 1½ cup catsup.

DIRECTIONS

1. Bring a bowl and combine all of the ingredients together. Mix well and cover the bowl.

2. Add to the fridge to set for half an hour or more.

3. Serve with your favorite seafood options.

NUTRITION (per serving): Calories: 56 kcal | Fats: 0g | Carbs: 14g | Protein: 0g.

144. LOW-SUGAR BBQ SAUCE

 0 min

 50 min

 Sauces & Seasonings

 4 Servings

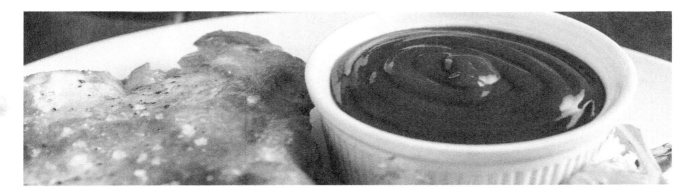

INGREDIENTS

- 1 tbsp. olive oil
- 1 large, sweet onion, chopped
- 4 garlic cloves, minced
- 1½ cups Heinz low sugar ketchup
- 1½ cups tomato sauce
- ¼ cup vinegar
- ½ cup Splenda Brown Sugar
- 2 tbsp. lemon juice
- 4 tbsp. brown mustard
- 2 tbsp. Worcestershire sauce
- 1 tsp. salt
- ½ tsp. black pepper
- 5 tbsp. chili powder
- 2 tbsp. Liquid Smoke.

DIRECTIONS

1. Sauté the onion and garlic in olive oil over medium high heat until golden brown and softened.

2. Reduce heat to low and add ketchup, tomato sauce, vinegar, Splenda, lemon juice, mustard, Worcestershire sauce, salt, pepper, chili powder, and Liquid Smoke.

3. Simmer 30 to 45 minutes, until mixture is thick and delicious.

NUTRITION (per serving): Calories: 16 kcal | Fats: 0.2g | Carbs: 2.6g | Protein: 0g.

145. SUGAR FREE TERIYAKI SAUCE

10 min

0 min

Sauces & Seasonings

4 Servings

INGREDIENTS

- 1 cup soy sauce,
- ½ cup rice vinegar
- ½ cup Smucker's, sugar free (or low sugar orange marmalade)
- 1 tsp. garlic powder
- 1 tsp. freshly grated ginger
- ¼ tsp. red pepper flakes, crushed.

DIRECTIONS

1. Combine all ingredients in a small pan.

2. Warm mixture gently until melted.

3. Store in a small, covered container in the refrigerator until ready to use.

NUTRITION (per serving): Calories: 25 kcal | Fats: 1.8g | Carbs: 1.4g | Protein: 1.1g.

146. GREEK TZATZIKI

15 min

0 min

Sauces & Seasonings

4 Servings

INGREDIENTS

- 1 medium English cucumber
- 1 cup Greek whole milk yogurt
- 2 garlic cloves, finely minced
- 1 tsp. lemon zest
- 1 tbsp. fresh lemon juice
- 2 tbsp. fresh dill, chopped
- Salt and black pepper.

DIRECTIONS

1. Peel and grate the cucumber into a medium bowl - gather up into your hands and squeeze out a good amount of the excess water into a bowl or sink to discard.

2. In a medium bowl, whisk together the yogurt, cucumber, garlic, lemon zest, lemon juice and dill.

3. Season with 1 teaspoon salt and 1/2 teaspoon pepper and add more to your taste.

NUTRITION (per serving): Calories: 34 kcal | Fats: 1.2g | Carbs: 0.5g | Protein: 0.1g.

147. ITALIAN TOMATO SAUCE

 0 min

 20 min

 Sauces & Seasonings

 4 Servings

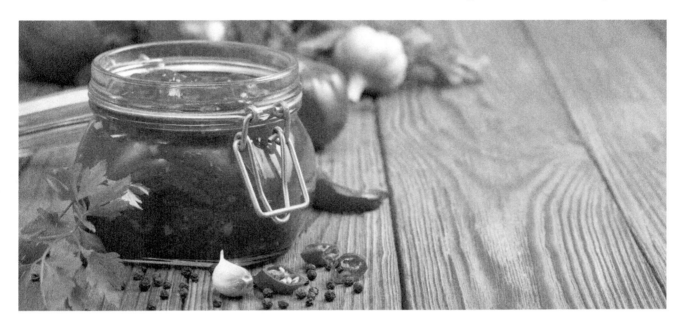

INGREDIENTS

- 3 tbsp. olive oil
- 1 large onion, finely chopped
- 5 garlic cloves, very thinly sliced
- 2 tbsp. dried basil
- 1/2 cup water (or white wine)
- ½ tsp. dried oregano
- ⅛ tsp. crushed red pepper
- 2 (28-ounce) cans crushed tomatoes
- 1½ tsp. salt
- ½ tsp. black pepper.

DIRECTIONS

1. Heat the olive oil in a medium saucepan over medium high heat and sauté the onion and garlic until softened and translucent.

2. Add the basil, oregano and red pepper and cook for one minute while stirring to infuse flavor into the olive oil.

3. Add the tomatoes, water (or white wine), salt and black pepper.

4. Lower heat to medium and bubble for 15 minutes.

NUTRITION (per serving): Calories: 31 kcal | Fats: 2.3g | Carbs: 4g | Protein: 0g.

148. ENCHILADA SAUCE

15 min	0 min	Sauces & Seasonings	2 Servings

INGREDIENTS

- 1 tomato, chopped
- ½ cup water
- 1 cup vegetable broth
- 1 tsp ground cumin
- ½ tsp. smoked paprika
- ½ tsp. dried oregano
- 1 tbsp. chili powder
- 2 tbsp. pastry flour
- 1 tsp. garlic, minced
- ¼ cup onion, chopped
- 2 tbsp. olive oil.

DIRECTIONS

1. Bring out a pan and heat it up on the stove. Add the garlic, onion, and oil and cook for a few minutes.

2. After this time, add the flour and then stir to make the garlic and onion get coated well.

3. Now add in the cumin, paprika, oregano, and chili powder. Then whisk in the water and broth, making sure to whisk often to avoid lumps.

4. Add in the tomatoes and cook until they start to thicken quite a bit. After this time, add all of this into an immersion blender until it is smooth.

5. When this is done, use it right away or store in an airtight container to use later.

NUTRITION (per serving): Calories: 37 kcal | Fats: 0g | Carbs: 7g | Protein: 0g.

Chapter 15

DESSERTS RECIPES

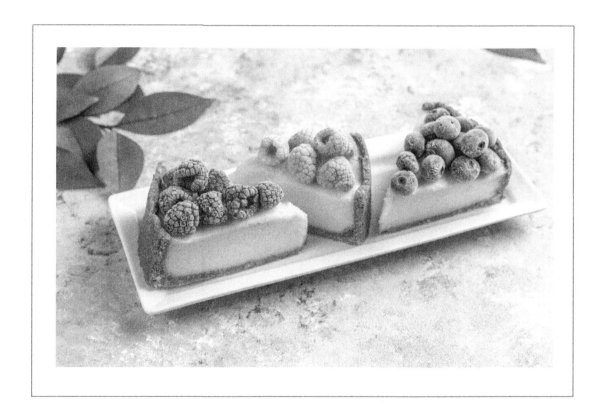

149. LOW SUGAR ICE CREAM CAKE

 2 h 15 min   10 min   Desserts   4-6 Servings

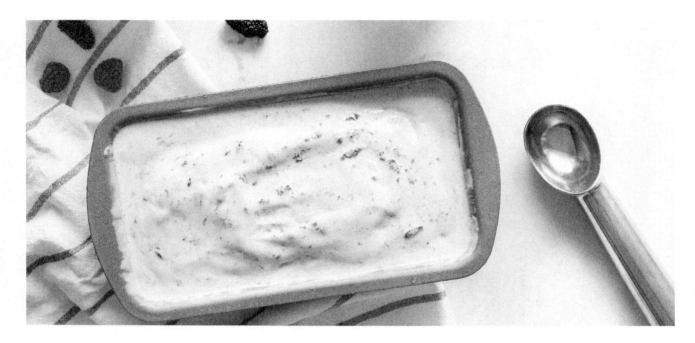

INGREDIENTS

- 1¼ cup of 1 or 2% milk
- 1 (4-serving) package Jello Sugar Free Instant Pudding mix - Vanilla flavor
- ½ tsp. vanilla
- 1 tsp. freshly grated lemon zest
- ½ lemon juice
- 1 (8-ounce) container regular Cool Whip, thawed
- ½ pint fresh raspberries.

DIRECTIONS

1. Line a loaf pan with plastic wrap and set aside.

2. Whisk the milk into the pudding mix in a medium bowl until smooth and thick. Stir in the vanilla, lemon zest and lemon juice.

3. Mix in half the Cool Whip to lighten mixture.

4. Gently fold in the remaining Cool Whip and then the berries.

5. Transfer to prepared loaf pan - fold wrap over top of 'cake' and place in level area of freezer. Freeze for 2 hours or until solid.

6. To serve: remove from freezer and allow to icy thaw for 15 minutes. Slice, garnish and serve!

NUTRITION (per serving): Calories: 115 kcal | Fats: 6.2g | Carbs: 13.7g | Protein: 1.3g.

150. PEAR-CRANBERRY PIE WITH OATMEAL STREUSEL

10 min

1 h

Desserts

6 Servings

INGREDIENTS

- ¾ cup oats
- ⅓ cup Stevia
- ½ tsp. cinnamon
- ¼ tsp. nutmeg
- 1 tbsp. butter, cubed

DIRECTIONS

1. Set oven to 350°F.
2. Combine all streusel ingredients in a food processor and process into a coarse crumb. Next, combine all filling ingredients in a large bowl and toss to combine. Transfer filling into pie crust, then top with streusel mix.
3. Set to bake until golden brown, about 1 hour. Cool and serve.

NUTRITION (per serving): Calories: 280 kcal | Fats: 9g | Carbs: 47g | Protein: 8g.

151. SUGAR FREE MOCHA CREAM

10 min

0 min

Desserts

2 Servings

INGREDIENTS

- 1 cup part-skim ricotta cheese
- 1 tsp. sugar-free cocoa powder
- ½ tsp. Espresso powder, or instant coffee granules
- ¼ tsp. vanilla extract
- 1 tbsp. Stevia
- 2 tsp. sugar-free mini chocolate chips, or finely chopped sugar-free chocolate.

DIRECTIONS

1. In a bowl mix together the ricotta, cocoa powder, espresso powder, vanilla extract, Stevia.
2. Divide into dessert bowls and garnish with chocolate.
3. Serve chilled.

NUTRITION (per serving): Calories: 238 kcal | Fats: 23.6g | Carbs: 11g | Protein: 2.8g.

152. PUMPKIN PIE SPICED YOGURT

15 min

0 min

Desserts

2 Servings

INGREDIENTS

- 2 cup low-fat plain yogurt
- ½ cup pumpkin puree
- ¼ tsp. cinnamon
- ¼ tsp. pumpkin pie spice
- ¼ cup chopped walnuts
- 1 tbsp. honey.

DIRECTIONS

1. Combine spices with the pumpkin puree in a medium bowl and stir.

2. Stir in yogurt, divide into 2 serving glasses. Top with honey and walnuts. Serve and enjoy!

NUTRITION (per serving): Calories: 207 kcal | Fats: 7g | Carbs: 22g | Protein: 6g.

153. TROPICAL DREAMS PUDDING

10 min

0 min

Desserts

4 Servings

INGREDIENTS

- 1 package sugar-free fat-free banana instant pudding mix
- 2 cups cold skim milk
- 4 scoops tropical fruit-flavored low-carb whey protein isolate powder.

DIRECTIONS

1. In a medium bowl, beat pudding mix, milk, and protein powder with an electric hand mixer until thoroughly blended and slightly thickened, about 2 minutes.

2. Pour pudding into 4 small bowls and refrigerate until set, about 5 minutes.

3. Serve immediately or cover and refrigerate for up to 2 days. Enjoy!

NUTRITION (per serving): Calories:125 kcal | Fats: 10g | Carbs: 12g | Protein: 7g.

154. NO BAKE STRAWBERRY CHEESECAKE

2 h 20 min

0 min

Desserts

6-8 Servings

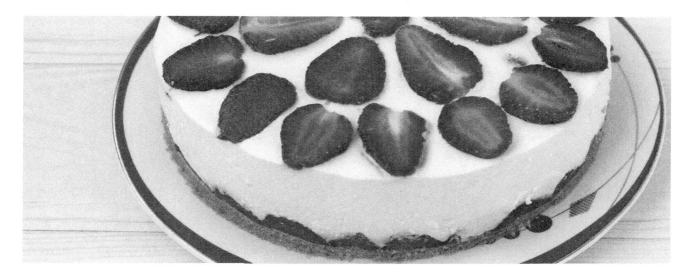

INGREDIENTS

- 8 oz. low- fat cream cheese, softened - do not use fat free
- ½ cup Stevia
- ½ cup sugar free strawberry preserves
- 1 (6-oz.) cup 2% Greek yogurt
- 1 tsp. vanilla extract
- 2 cups Cool Whip, thawed
- ¼ cup fresh strawberries, hulled and diced
- 5-6 strawberries to slice and decorate top of pie
- 2/3 package oatmeal cookies
- 1 tbsp. melted butter.

DIRECTIONS

1. For cookie crumb crust: pulse 2/3 package oatmeal cookies with 1 tablespoon melted butter in food processor and press into pie plate or springform bottom.

2. Beat the cream cheese and Stevia, using an electric mixer, until fluffy.

3. Add the preserves, yogurt and vanilla; beat until just combined.

4. Fold in the whipped topping and chopped strawberries.

5. Pile the filling into crust, smooth and either chill or freeze.

6. Remove from freezer about 20 minutes before serving to soften.

7. Arrange berry slices to decorate pie.

NUTRITION (per serving): Calories: 120 kcal | Fats: 2.1g | Carbs: 15.5g | Protein: 4.6g.

155. TENDER PEACH COBBLER

 15 min

 40 min

 Desserts

 6-8 Servings

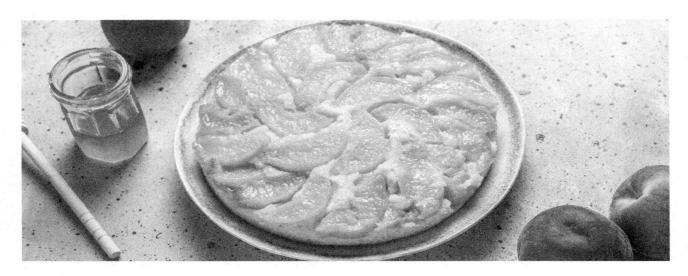

INGREDIENTS

- 4 tbsp. butter
- 1 cup all-purpose flour
- ½ cup Stevia
- 1½ tsp. baking powder
- ¼ tsp. salt
- 1 cup milk
- 2 (14-ounce) cans no added sugar peach slices
- Ground cinnamon.

DIRECTIONS

1. Preheat oven to 325°F.

2. Melt butter by slicing and arranging in an 8-inch square ceramic baking dish placed in oven while heating - set aside.

3. Combine flour, Stevia, baking powder, salt and slowly add milk while mixing to avoid lumps.

4. Pour mixture over melted butter - do not stir.

5. Using a large spoon, scoop fruit directly from the cans over the top of the batter - point is to scoop them with some of the liquid from the can.

6. Sprinkle with cinnamon. Batter will rise to top during baking.

7. Bake 30 to 40 minutes, until golden and pick inserted near center has moist crumb but fairly clean.

8. Serve warm.

NUTRITION (per serving): Calories: 165.5 kcal | Fats: 3.7g | Carbs: 27.6g | Protein: 2.7g.

156. SUGAR FREE COCONUT CAKE

15 min

45 min

Desserts

6-8 Servings

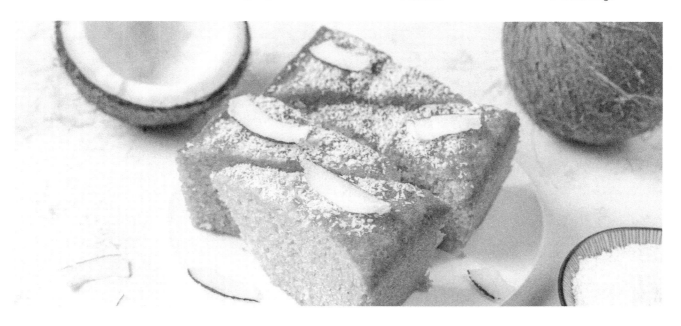

INGREDIENTS

- 1 cup all-purpose flour
- ½ cup almond flour
- ¼ cup unsweetened coconut
- ½ cup Stevia
- 1 tsp. baking soda
- ½ tsp. salt
- 1 cup milk
- 4 tbsp. butter, melted
- 1 tsp. pure vanilla extract
- 1 tsp. coconut extract
- 1 tbsp. apple cider vinegar.

DIRECTIONS

1. Preheat oven to 375°F. Lightly coat 8-inch round cake pan with cooking spray and set aside.

2. In a large bowl whisk together flour, almond flour, coconut, Stevia, baking soda, and salt. In a small bowl whisk together the milk, butter and extracts. Add the liquids to the dry, blending until smooth. Stir in the vinegar.

3. Pour into prepared pan and bake until center springs back, 30 to 35 minutes.

4. Cool 10 minutes before turning onto rack to cool completely. Cut into thin wedges and serve with fruit or a small scoop of sugar free vanilla ice cream.

NUTRITION (per serving): Calories: 198 kcal | Fats: 6.9g | Carbs: 36.6g | Protein: 2.3g.

157. CARROT CAKE - NO SUGAR ADDED

15 min

35 min

Desserts

6-8 Servings

The cake is super moist, delicious and completely 'no added sugar' as its very lightly sweetened with stevia. It does have calories and carbs, so have a small slice.

INGREDIENTS

- ¾ cup almond flour
- ¾ cup all-purpose flour
- 1½ tsp. baking powder
- ½ tsp. salt
- 1 tsp. ground cinnamon
- ½ tsp. ground cardamom
- ½ cup Stevia
- 3 large eggs
- ½ cup plain yogurt or sour cream, reduced fat
- 1 tsp. vanilla
- 4 tbsp. butter, melted
- 3 medium carrots, grated

<u>FROSTING INGREDIENTS</u>

- 4 oz. Philadelphia light cream cheese (not fat free)
- 1 cup heavy cream or whipping cream
- 1 tbsp. Jello Sugar Free Instant Vanilla Pudding powder
- ¼ cup finely chopped walnuts.

DIRECTIONS

1. Preheat oven to 350°F.

2. Spray an 8-inch round cake pan with vegetable cooking spray and line with a round of parchment or waxed paper.

3. Blend the almond flour, flour, baking powder, salt, cinnamon and cardamom in a medium bowl and set aside.

4. Whisk the Stevia, eggs, yogurt, vanilla and butter in a large bowl until creamy; add the dry ingredients and mix until just blended. Fold in the carrots.

5. Pour into prepared pan and bake 30 to 35 minutes until toothpick inserted near center comes out clean. Turn out onto cooling rack and peel off paper.

6. If making the topping: whip cream cheese until fluffy, add cream and pudding powder and beat until smooth and creamy.

7. When cake is completely cooled, scrape frosting onto center of layer, spread to edges and level.

8. Sprinkle with the walnuts.

9. Chill until serving.

NUTRITION (per serving): Calories: 210.7 kcal | Fats: 8.9g | Carbs: 24.7g | Protein: 5.6g.

158. NO SUGAR ADDED BROWNIES

 15 min

 25 min

 Desserts

 16 Servings

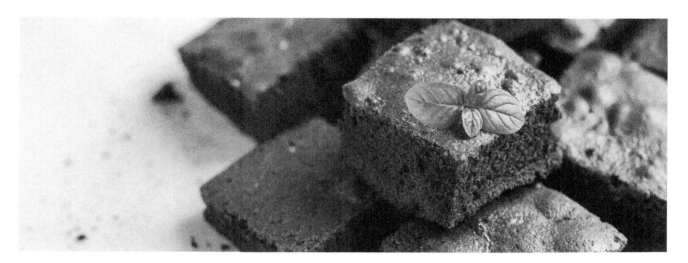

INGREDIENTS

- Vegetable cooking spray
- 1 (15-ounce) can black beans, well rinsed and drained
- ½ cup Stevia
- 3 tbsp. butter, melted
- 1 tsp. vanilla
- 3 large eggs
- ½ cup Dutch cocoa - smoother, richer, less bitter
- ½ tsp. Espresso powder, or instant coffee granules
- ½ tsp. baking powder
- ½ tsp. salt
- ½ cup sugar free or dark chocolate, chopped.

DIRECTIONS

1. Preheat oven to 350°F.

2. Spray an 8x8-inch baking dish with vegetable oil cooking spray.

3. Puree the black beans in food processor until fairly smooth.

4. Scrape down sides and add Stevia, butter, vanilla and one egg. Process until very smooth.

5. Scrape down sides and add 2 remaining eggs, cocoa, coffee, baking powder, salt and chopped chocolate.

6. Process until well blended, scraping down sides and processing to a creamy batter.

7. Pour batter into prepared pan and bake until toothpick inserted 2 inches from center tests done, 18 to 25 minutes.

8. Cool completely before cutting into two-inch squares.

NUTRITION (per serving): Calories: 179 kcal | Fats: 9.2g | Carbs: 10.2g | Protein: 17.3g.

159. LOW-CARB LEMON BARS

25 min

30 min

Desserts

12 Servings

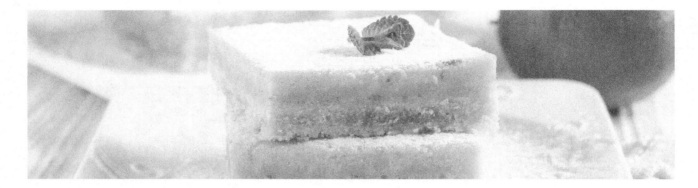

INGREDIENTS

FILLING
- 8 lemons juiced
- 1 cup liquid egg substitute
- 3 egg yolks
- ¾ cup Stevia
- 1 tbsp. corn starch

CRUST
- 1 cup high fiber cereal
- 1 cup coconut flour
- 2 tbsp. Stevia
- 5 oz. low-fat cream cheese softened
- Pinch salt.

DIRECTIONS

1. Preheat oven to 350°F.

2. In a bowl, mix together cereal, coconut flour, sweetener and salt. Add softened cream cheese and mix until it forms a clumpy sand-like mixture that can form into a loose ball in your hand.

3. Line an 8x8-inch baking pan with parchment paper, then press the crumb mixture into it. Bake the crust 15 minutes, then allow it to cool.

4. In a mixing bowl, combine lemon juice, liquid egg substitute, egg yolks and sweetener. Whisk thoroughly or beat with a hand mixer on medium speed. Add cornstarch and mix thoroughly again.

5. Pour lemon mixture over crust and set the entire baking dish on the bottom rack of your oven. Bake for 25-30 minutes or until the lemon custard is just set.

6. Allow to cool thoroughly before removing the entire recipe from the baking dish using the parchment paper. Cut into squares and refrigerate in an airtight container until ready to eat.

NUTRITION (per serving): Calories: 166 kcal | Fats: 12.7g | Carbs: 5g | Protein: 6g.

Printed in Great Britain
by Amazon